the joy of keeping

farm
animals

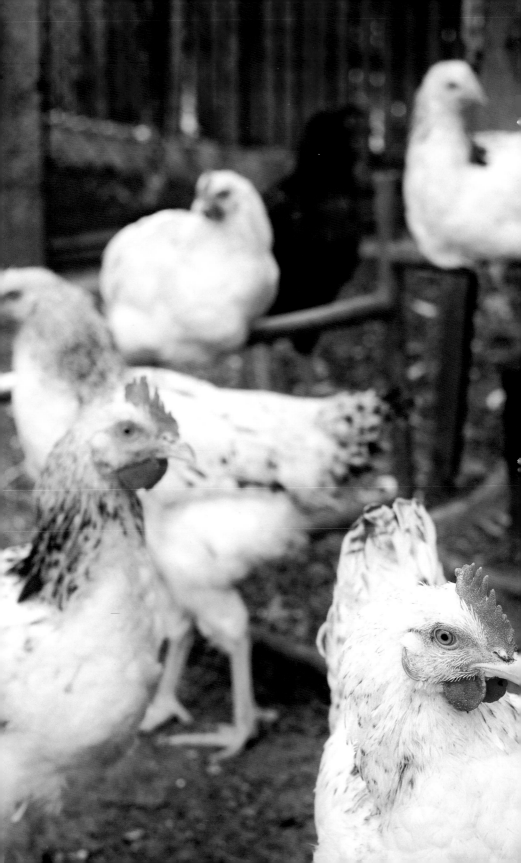

SECOND EDITION

the joy of keeping

farm animals

RAISING CHICKENS, GOATS, PIGS, SHEEP, AND COWS

Laura Childs

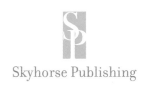

Skyhorse Publishing

Skyhorse Publishing books may be purchased in bulk at special discounts for sales promotion, corporate gifts, fund-raising, or educational purposes. Special editions can also be created to specifications. For details, contact the Special Sales Department, Skyhorse Publishing, 307 West 36th Street, 11th Floor, New York, NY 10018 or info@skyhorsepublishing.com.

Skyhorse® and Skyhorse Publishing® are registered trademarks of Skyhorse Publishing, Inc.®, a Delaware corporation.

Visit our website at www.skyhorsepublishing.com.

The information in this book is true and complete to the best of the author's knowledge. This book is not intended to be a substitute for veterinary care, and all the recipes and instructions for food preparation are to be used at your own risk. The author and publisher make all recommendations without guarantee, and disclaim any liability arising in connection with this information.

10 9 8 7 6 5 4 3 2

Library of Congress Cataloging-in-Publication Data

Childs, Laura, 1963-
The joy of keeping farm animals : Raising Chickens, Goats, Pigs, Sheep, and Cows / Laura Childs.
p. cm.
Includes index.
(pbk. : alk. paper)
1. Livestock farms. 2. Domestic animals. 3. Animal products.
4. Food animals. I. Title.
SF65.2.C45 2010
636—dc22
2009034217

Cover design by LeAnna Weller Smith
Cover photos from Shutterstock.com

Print ISBN: 978-1-63220-468-4
Ebook ISBN: 978-1-63450-125-5

Printed in China

Goodbye my Kizzy.
I miss you already.

contents

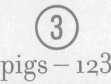
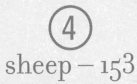

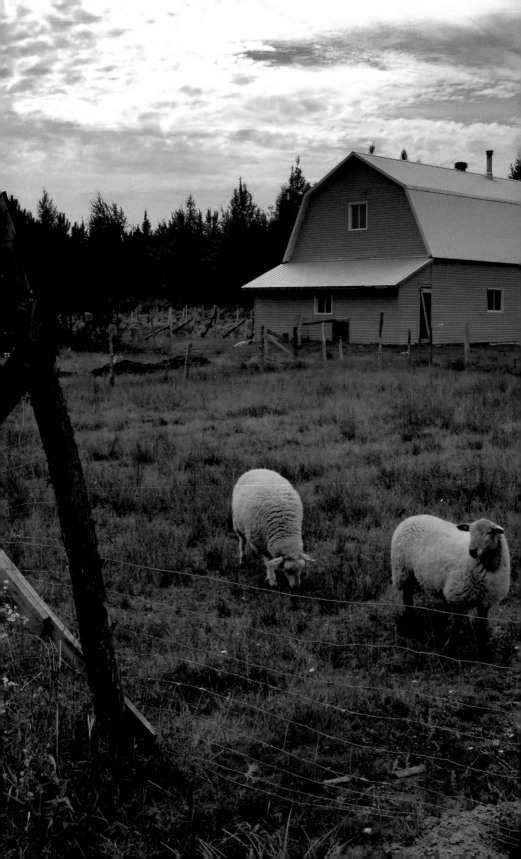

preface

Wide open spaces and sunny front porches. A little garden, a little barn, and a few animals scattering the landscape.

Therein lies the romanticism of a life in the country.

This was the life I yearned to provide for my daughter. The opportunity to grow up on the basics, away from chaos and unreasonable schedules.

A place to ponder, to find purpose and meaning. To better understand our Earth and her inhabitants. To recognize our reliance on things that can't be plugged into a wall socket.

I had lived for years in the center of a large metropolis. While I had loved every minute of it, I knew that I would have neither means nor time enough to connect my daughter to the world around us.

After two wide right turns from the highway and a few minutes of travel along a dirt road, we came to the end of a long overgrown driveway; there our journey began.

I was a single mother with no idea how to grow a zucchini, much less nurture the tender spirit of a three-year-old child.

For the first few months I felt like Eva Gabor's character in the late 1960s sitcom *Green Acres*. I connected so deeply to her that I even started a website called *Good Bye City Life* with plans to chronicle our upcoming misadventures. Those high-end boots and designer labels just weren't built for barn chores.

The local folk watched us arrive, learned that we had no nearby relatives, and made secret bets on how soon the old place would be back up for sale.

Seventeen years passed.

A child was raised and raised well. Together, we grew most of our own food. Through love and toil and occasional sadness we learned the invaluable power of self-reliance.

In full disclosure, we were never completely alone. As trite as the earlier bets had seemed, many watched over and prayed for us. We were lucky to possess the two most revered traits in a rural community—pure grit and humble spirit.

Of the two, humility—or lack of pretentiousness—was the true key to survival. To ask for and accept advice, assistance, and trust—without posturing or flaunting past city life accomplishments—serves new homesteaders well. When you have nothing to prove, country folk welcome and accept you with open arms.

In her sixteenth year, Veronica and I conferred over this book's approach. Keeping farm animals, we've decided, is a balancing act of joy and morality. The ethics of animal husbandry, the environmental impact of every step, and eating well will be discoveries that depend on your personal comfort zone.

This book does contain information on keeping farm animals with the intent of feeding your family. The alternative (aside from being a vegetarian) is to purchase pristine white packages of meat from the grocery store—the meat of animals that quite likely had a miserable life, or at the very least a miserable end. The mainstream media has effectively shattered our trust in commercially harvested food.

Country wisdom overrides sentimentality within the remainder of these pages but it must be said that sentencing an animal to the dinner table is a certainly a somber act. My advice is to do so with the utmost appreciation and gratitude, and with all the dignity your animals deserve—this will be your redemption as you provide for your family.

Raise what you can as best you can. Keep your humble spirit about you. Count every step of good stewardship as a joy and you will be richly rewarded.

acknowledgments

The credit for content herein goes to my daughter Veronica. She carried me to this land and worked at my side to explore the joys, hard work, and wonders of raising farm animals and growing our own food. To think it all began with a tiny pack of carrot seeds and some really cute gardening gloves! "Let's do it together, Mom."

Although I have been the fingers at the keyboard, not one word of this book would have been possible without the cocreation and collaboration of ideals and understanding from a long list of supportive friends, old-time farmers, and personal resources. Special thanks to Don and Shelley Douglas, Erin Neese, Jennifer and Curtis Foster, David and Lucille Burke, David and Diane Peck, Richard and Julie Koster, Linda Ann Hart and Drew Freymond, my budding list of photographers, and the thousands of subscribers who have e-mailed accounts of their own adventures in farm life for the past ten years via GoodByeCityLife.com

To Ann Treistman, who repeatedly challenged and graciously assisted me in the personal adventure of writing a book for print publication. Thanks also to the rest of the team at Skyhorse Publishing: Tony Lyons, Bill Wolfsthal, Abigail Gehring, Cat Kovach, Ashley Albert, and last but not least, designer LeAnna Weller Smith.

A very special thanks to my candid husband of the last six years, Eric Kleinoder. Without him I would have brought every animal into the house when temperatures dipped below freezing and spent my life savings on raising pigs, chickens, goats, and sheep well past their point of value. Pugnaciousness aside and without judgment, today he'll gently smile while he trips over the orphaned calf spending a few nights in our laundry room and the broody hen nesting in the basement. One important lesson I've learned from Eric, one which every new and tenderhearted farmer needs to at least partially understand, is: "These animals may be intelligent, may show appreciation and acceptance of their keeper, but it is a mistake to put every human emotion on an animal."

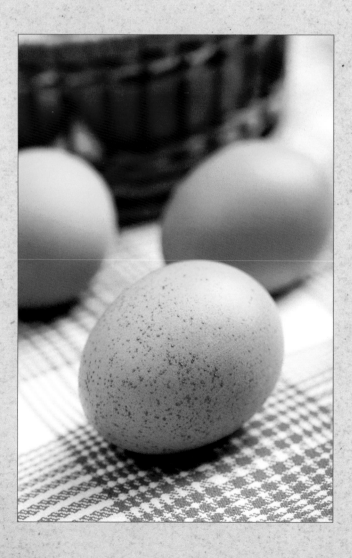

introduction

Some of the most memorable and rewarding experiences can be found in keeping barnyard animals.

To awake in the morning by the rooster's crow.

To gaze outside your breakfast window, watching sheep in their peaceful graze of green pastures.

Even to be called to the chores of their keep—work so slight when measured against the return. On the way to the barnyard, you pause just long enough to wonder why life took you down the long road to get here.

The joy found in keeping farm animals isn't a one-dimensional foray into raising a healthier food source. The joy is in fact multi-layered, ever evolving, and inspirational. Through tending to a small group of barnyard guests you'll discover new appreciation for Earth and all of her inhabitants, a discernment between morality and profit, and a desire to take responsible action for the sake of future generations.

Keeping farm animals is a sharp contrast to our high-tech, low-touch, modern life. The start of each new day is no longer spent at a computerized device checking texts and replying to e-mails. Instead you will be called upon to partake in a hands-on, rewarding experience. You can fill up the hours between morning and evening chores with all the business and bother of an average modern day, but those trappings are soon to be sandwiched by the joy of pastures, coops, and barnyards.

Benefits to keeping farm animals are greater still if you have children in your life. Learning and exploring the complexity of different animals with an adult is a bonding exercise a child will never forget.

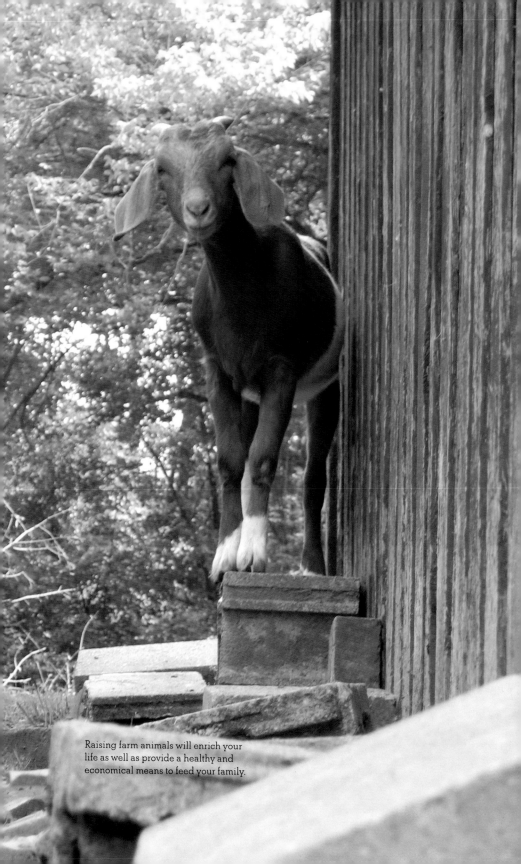

Raising farm animals will enrich your life as well as provide a healthy and economical means to feed your family.

Children who have taken part in raising farm animals understand the process of procreation, experience the miracle of birth, and appreciate each meal placed before them in ways that many in this world cannot—even the vast majority of adults who have never contemplated the life that existed previous to the tidy white supermarket package. Ask any country child, however, and you'll receive a systematic walk-through of the most probable journey from barn to table.

A Change of Heart

At a time in our lives when we don't think we can take on one more daily task or chore, the act of keeping farm animals may seem daunting. Others have passed this way before and I have been one of them. I assure you there is time enough in all our lives for the amount of chores any farm animal within the pages of this book requires.

In time you won't be counting chores as added responsibility, but as a labor of love.

Love?

Yes. In a noble and caring admiration of those you keep. If there is but one inherent trait of every happy backyard farmer I've crossed paths with—no matter how busy their lives—it is that they love the animals they keep, even though surface intention might appear otherwise. With honor and with tender compassion they find joy in the effort expended tending to their own food source, knowing the value of doing so and sharing the bounty with friends and family.

Preparation and Practicality

Keeping any animal—farm or pet—requires knowledge as well as time. The very fact that you've picked up and are reading this book is a signal of the highest intention—to gain wisdom enough to provide the best possible life for the food animals you raise, no matter how short their stay on your land may be.

Apart from providing basic care, other preliminary questions may arise. Below are a few questions to which you'll want to have answers before you begin setting up for or bringing home new animals.

- Do local zoning regulations allow this animal on my property?
- Do I have a backup plan or person to help with chores if I am called away or get sick?
- What will I do with the offspring if my animals breed?
- What is my plan for dealing with barnyard waste and manure?
- Who can I rely on for veterinary support? What if I need a veterinarian in the middle of the night or on a weekend?
- Does someone exist in my community or personal network who will answer questions for me on the health and maintenance of my chosen animal or breed?

Within these pages you will find insights into the very nature of each animal. Through understanding their instinctual nature you will be able to read their cycles, health levels, and needs.

RIGHT: The author's daughter, Veronica. At fifteen years old she still can't resist a trip to the livestock auction. Today she brings home a baby duck to raise, but past purchases have not been so easy to transport. The family rule, years in the making, is: "If you bring it home, you have to care for it yourself!"

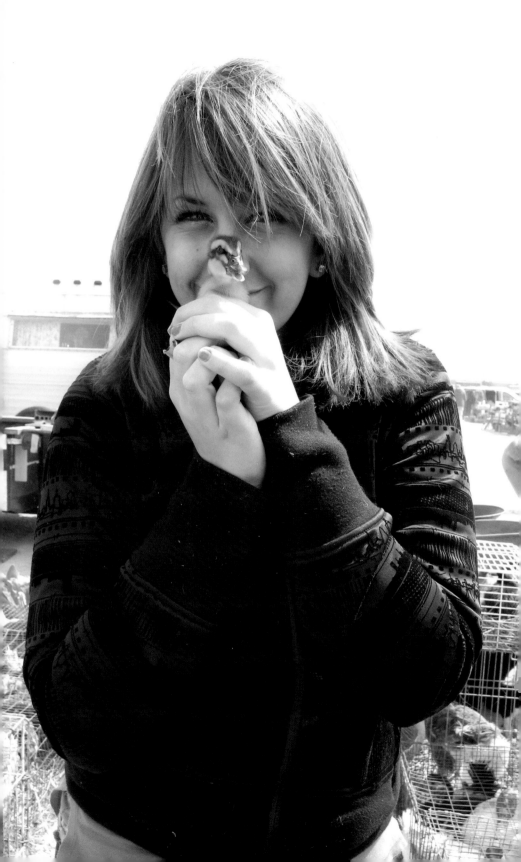

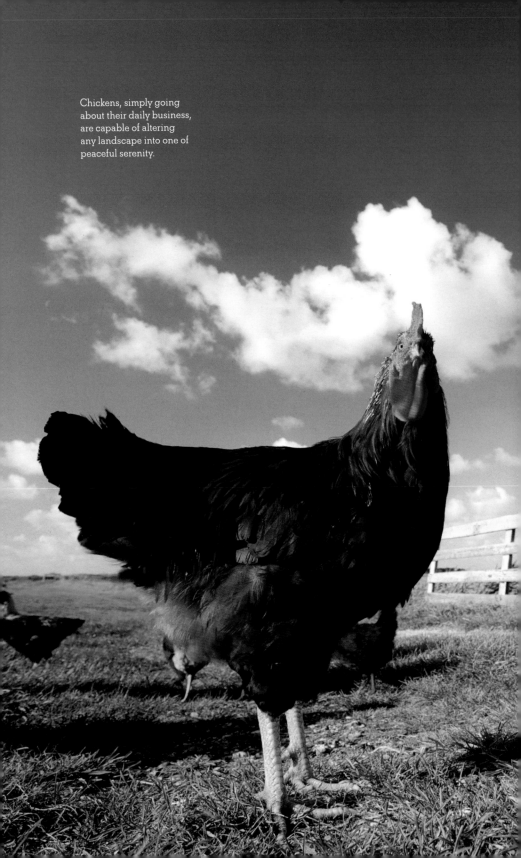

Chickens, simply going
about their daily business,
are capable of altering
any landscape into one of
peaceful serenity.

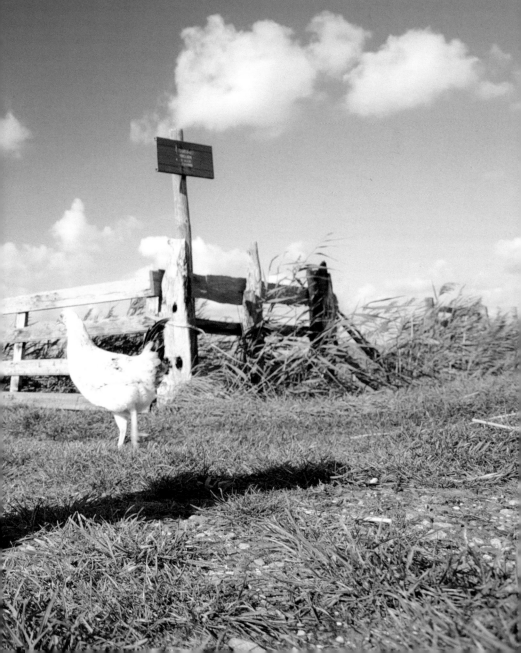

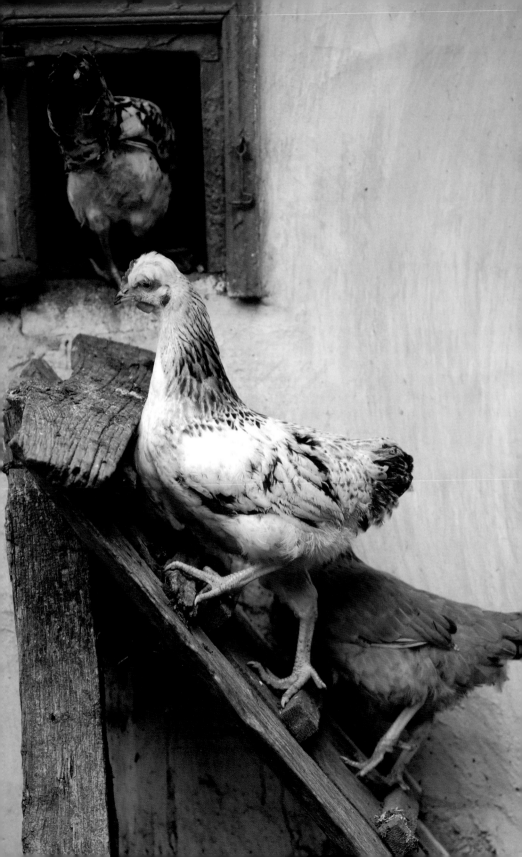

No farm animal typifies the country-living experience better than a chicken. A few scattered hens lazily picking through the grass, a rooster strutting along the fence rail, or the whole lot scurrying to the child who calls them in for grain—their very presence on the landscape stirs the romanticism of simpler times.

Psychological effects aside, the rewards of keeping chickens are numerous. They'll bless your home with the finest quality, the tastiest, and the healthiest eggs and poultry you have ever consumed.

Since early domestication, this is the way chicken and eggs were meant to be enjoyed. Your taste buds will be challenged to be satisfied with the grocer's version ever again.

Knowing that the food at home is superior in all regards, you may soon find yourself turning up your nose at restaurant and take-out meals.

Chickens are also an easy, inexpensive keep. Provided that you already have a small shed, you could be enjoying fresh eggs just a few days from now.

If I had but four sentences to describe the joy of keeping chickens they would be: "Cheap to purchase and to feed. Don't require much in way of housing. A few minutes per day to care for. Blessings unnumbered as reward." Where else can you get so much for so little?

Energy-Efficient Poultry

It takes:

Twenty pounds of feed to produce one pound of beef.

Three and one half pounds of feed to produce one pound of protein from eggs*.

Two pounds of feed to produce one pound of chicken.

* The average large egg contains 0.7 pounds of protein.

A Healthier Alternative for Your Family

Purchasing poultry and eggs at your local grocery store is a budget-friendly way to feed your family. Compared to an unknown risk—that raising chickens at home might cost more—you may wonder if the added responsibility is worth all the bother. Setting economics and household budgets aside for later discussion, I assure you that raising your own eggs and poultry is definitely worth the bother. What you don't pay for today at the grocery store, you may be paying for in the future with your health.

Commercially raised poultry and eggs are reasonably priced due to the volume and efficiency of chicken factories in North America. With highly efficient systems and rigorous demands, these factories have mastered the art of maximum output with minimal waste of labor, space, and feed. Although it may be admirable on the surface (their efficiency facilitates lower grocery bill totals for families), you can't help but wonder, "At what real cost?"

- Less flavor, nutrition, and freshness.
- Potentially more chemicals, residual antibiotics, unnatural hormones and additives to the end product.
- Our consumption of animals that have led miserable lives.

This is what we have been feeding, for the most part unaware, to our families, the effects and health risks of which are yet to be fully discovered.

Until now.

In the last fifteen years, there has been no escaping monthly news reports across the continent, health articles around the world, and feature film documentaries on the implications of production-raised poultry. Large-scale poultry growers and egg factories are fined or shut down regularly for unsanitary, inhumane, and unethical practices. Many more continue to operate unnoticed. Neither blowing the whistle nor passing judgment on every packing house or poultry factory, the following growing practices are more common in North America than we know.

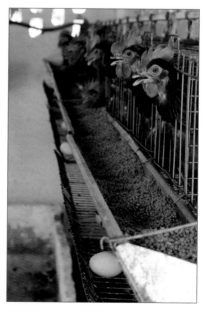

- Meat birds are being fed hormones for fast growth. To deal with unsanitary conditions and stress-related sickness brought on from overcrowding, they are also fed a steady diet of antibiotic-laden feed.

ABOVE: Red sex-link hens, confined from the age of twenty weeks, spend their lives eating and producing eggs in harsh conditions.

- Laying hens are restricted to cages barely larger than their
  own bodies, in rooms where lights are left on for twenty-
  four hours a day, fed production-inducing and antibiotic-
  laden feed, and then culled the very day they stop laying.

These are possibly the only avenues poultry and egg factory
farms have to feed a hungry, budget-conscious nation while still
turning a profit. Yet our increasing awareness of these practices
make inexpensive eggs and poultry seem less a bargain in the
checkout line.

There is a better way.

Growing your own chicken and keeping laying hens buys you
peace of mind. You know precisely the quality of the nourishment
you are setting upon your dinner table, the humane manner in
which that animal has been raised, and who you are supporting
through purchase.

The Challenges of Chickens

Raising your own poultry is personally satisfying, but the journey
from chick to table will have a few challenges along the way.

Although the positive aspects outweigh the negative, three
common annoyances are dust, smell, and noise. The latter two are
easily controlled. Dust, however, is inescapable.

Even a flock of ten chickens can create a considerable amount
of dust through their litter and dander. This, plus the possibility
of disease or virus transfer to other farm animals, is the primary
reason poultry should have their own shelter.

A substantial portion of your coop chores will be based on dust
removal. As long as the chickens are self-contained and healthy, it
is your personal choice either to manage it regularly or to delegate
the task to a larger, quarterly cleaning. As you've protected other
farm animals from poultry dust, don't neglect yourself during coop
cleaning. Wear a surgical mask, or even a kerchief over your nose
and mouth, to avoid inhalation of the fine dust. Lung health implications of poultry dust are well-documented as cumulative.

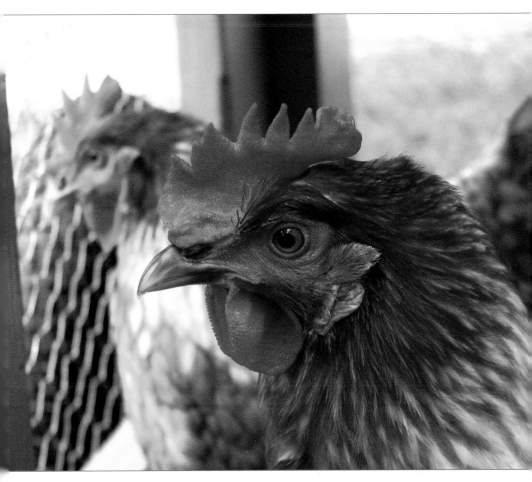

ABOVE: To keep all animals on your farm protected, chickens should have their own shelter.

The final two challenges, smell and noise, are often neighborly complaints. Sharing your farm-fresh eggs across the fence will go a long way to keeping the peace. If your coop is located on a shared property line, add a little extra litter to dramatically reduce coop odors, and avert potential noise complaints by opting out of keeping a rooster. A rooster's crow begins at the very first show of light, continues throughout the day, and can carry for a mile or more. Unless you are planning on breeding your laying hens and hatching out chicks, the rooster is nothing more than pretty plumage.

Choosing a Breed to Raise

Knowing your objective for raising chickens is the first step to selecting a breed that is right for you. While some breeds have been developed for maximum egg production, others excel at quick growth and efficient feed conversion. Chicken breeds are therefore classified as egg layers, meat birds, or dual-purpose. A final class, the exhibition breeds, are beautiful and useful but are not considered top producers for home farms. For your time, space, and money, the first three classifications provide the highest return on investment.

The list of chicken breeds to choose from is extensive. On GoodByeCityLife.com I maintain an ever-growing list of over one hundred known breeds, and I have only scratched the surface. All reputable hatcheries produce catalogs of the most popular breeds for your region, as well as a few fancy and hatchery-developed hybrids. Within each description you'll discover the hardiness, expected size, and production rates of each breed offered.

CHICKEN FUNDAMENTALS

Although a few breeds' needs vary in particularity, chickens all require three commonalities in care:
- A commitment to a chore schedule that keeps their coop and equipment clean.
- Access to fresh water and feed at all times.
- Safety from disease, weather extremes, and predators.

Egg Layers

The egg-laying breeds have been developed to provide maximum egg output from the smallest feed intake. Although the hens of these breeds perform best in the controlled environments of large-scale farming, their

ABOVE: Should you choose production over personality, the White Leghorn is considered a top layer in her class. These hens are high strung and seldom bond with their keepers, but their feed-to-egg ability is unmatched.

small-farm use is popular with families looking only for a supply of fresh eggs. Supplementary heat and lighting ensures healthy hens provide a steady supply of eggs in regions where temperatures drop below 60 degrees Fahrenheit.

Hens in this class will lay six to seven eggs per week for two years. By their third year, output is decreased to 50 percent or less and the hens are considered spent. Hens are small and the meat can be tough but may be sufficient to flavor a small soup.

The Productive Life of a Laying Hen

A pullet (female chicken) will have eaten twenty-five pounds of feed before she begins laying at twenty to twenty-four weeks.

At thirty weeks she will produce a standard-size egg almost daily.

At seventy-five weeks of age she will go through a molting period (replacing old feathers with new) for approximately eight weeks. During the molt she may not produce at all.

In her first laying year she will supply about twenty dozen eggs. In her second year her eggs will be larger but production will decrease to sixteen to eighteen dozen eggs per year. By the third year she is considered a spent hen and may only lay one egg every three to four days.

Meat Breeds

Very few North Americans raise a pure meat breed for the freezer, opting instead to raise a faster-growing cross. The most popular and easy-to-grow cross is that of a Cornish game (a true meat breed) with the Plymouth Rock (a dual-purpose breed) for its excellence in feed-to-meat conversion. A good cross will eat two pounds of feed for every pound of weight gained. By nine weeks of age the conversion ratio begins to deteriorate.

The drawback to growing these crosses is that they can neither be bred nor kept long-term. Each time you need to replenish your freezer's supply of poultry you'll be back at the hatchery placing another order.

Dual-Purpose Breeds

It is in this class you will find the breeds that fulfill the romanticism of country life, as well as the needs of a small farm or homestead. All dual-purpose breeds produce and grow at similar rates, have interesting personalities, and are easily trained. If your goal is to become self-sufficient, you could order a rooster to match your hens and eliminate future hatchery orders.

Early American settlers developed the most common of these breeds, producing weather-hardy laying hens and cockerels that grow to broiler size.

Although not as efficient at feed conversion as a meat breed cross, the dual-purpose cockerel finishes as a delicious three-pound meal for your dinner table by eighteen weeks. The hens, most of which you'll keep for two years, produce 75 to 80 percent of a dedicated egg-laying breed's volume.

The oldest and most popular breeds in this class are the Plymouth Rock, the Rhode Island Red, the Delaware, and the New Hampshire. Hatchery-specific hybrids and crosses are also popular in this class and are offered under a variety of names. As an example the common Red Sex Link or Red Star (or any other name a hatchery deems marketable) is created by breeding a dual-purpose Rhode Island Red rooster to a laying-breed Leghorn hen. The resulting hens are hardier than the Leghorn and have a higher egg production than the pure Rhode Island Red. The resulting cockerels, however, have a slightly smaller finishing weight than a pure Rhode Island Red.

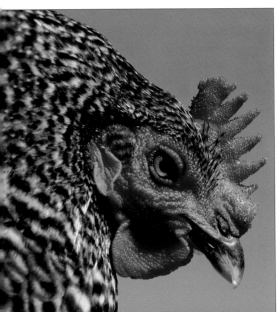

LEFT: The Barred Plymouth Rock, developed in America. A proficient dual-purpose layer that also grows to broiler size by twenty weeks of age.

Chicken Instinct and Temperament

Chickens, an easy keep and simple in needs, have quirks and instinctual oddities all their own. They'll make you laugh, contemplate the human complexity of life, and frustrate you all at the same time with their actions and antics.

Whether you want to train your chickens to come running when you call, break bad habits, or understand and work within the scope of their quirks, you'll need to understand their instincts and motivations.

Social Order in Flocks

Chickens have a highly developed social order. Starting with the rooster or lead hen and organized down to the weakest chick, every flock member has its place.

Chickens raised together will have established the flock's social order by three weeks of age.

Social order is maintained through pecking. The top hen can peck everyone, and the second hen can peck everyone except for the top hen, all the way down the line until the very last hen. She is pecked by all but cannot peck back. If you watch closely you can note which of your hens are lowest in the chain.

Whenever you introduce a new hen to the flock, the social order is disturbed. The resulting aggression is worthy of concern. Existing flocks have been known to kill a new hen in their effort to "put her in her place." New hens need slow introductions into established flocks. A fence between them for a week or two helps make the transition smoother. As an extra precaution, introduce the new hen to the others one at a time, beginning with the lowest in the pecking order.

Cocks are always prone to a hearty scrap, even after they seem to have reached an understanding. If they have accepted their places and established their own flocks of hens and feed stations, the need to squabble is lessened. Some cocks are more aggressive than others and may never accept another male in their vicinity.

Cannibalism and Feather Picking

The worst pecking habit is cannibalism. In the brooding box and under bright heat lamps, chicks begin to feather out. Their brood mates, noticing the new small specks appearing, peck at each other. Pecking escalates, one weaker chick is picked on, and eventually the entire flock is in on the action.

These chickens are, for the most part, bored. With exercise and a red heat lamp (red minimizes the show of new feathers), you can prevent this altogether. Provide low perches at various heights for one- to four-week-old chicks to keep them physically occupied.

Feather picking is similar to cannibalism. Hens will pull on their own feathers as well as others in the flock. Although it can be prevented with a beak trim at sixteen to twenty weeks, it is more important to determine the cause. Improper feed, unbalanced nutrients in the feed, bright lights for too many hours, poor ventilation in the coop, overcrowding, boredom, and parasitic infestation are all known causes of feather picking.

Egg Eating

Laying hens, coming of age, commonly drop their first eggs on the floor on their way to the nesting box. The egg may crack or the other hens may peck at the egg. Chickens find eggs tasty and as soon as this happens, the egg-eating habit has begun—not even eggs laid in the nest will be safe.

Knowledge serves prevention. Watch coming-of-age layers and never leave an egg on the floor—even if it's soiled and your hands are full. If you have many hens laying their eggs on the floor, check the dimensions and accessibility of the nesting boxes you've provided.

Training Chickens to Come

Chickens, like most any other animals, can be trained through food reward. Scratch grain is easily accessible. My hens' favorite treats are cheese and cantaloupe. When you're training chickens to come, use a key word or sound to trigger a treat or you'll have them rushing to you at every sighting.

Training takes no time at all and could save a chicken's life if you need to get him back to the coop in a hurry. For a few consecutive days, while they're all going about their business, start calling them with your trigger word and drop a little scratch grain on clean, dry ground. A few will come over to investigate. Flock mentality will soon have them all around your feet. Keep using the trigger word and keep dropping grain for four to five minutes. That's all there is to it.

The Need to Brood

The Little Red Hen's Gosling

A few years ago my mother goose repeatedly, systematically, and daily, rolled one egg out of her nest. I kept putting it back. She kept rolling it out. I could have taken it as a sign of natural selection. Instead I tucked the goose egg under a laying hen already nesting on her own eggs. The goose egg took longer than the others beneath her, but my Rhode Island Red hen still hatched and later mothered her gosling.

A hen's natural instinct is to lay a clutch of eggs, then sit on and hatch them. Yet every day you enter the coop and remove her egg, effectively returning her to day one of the process. If she has a very strong desire to brood, she might sit on and defend any egg she finds in the nest.

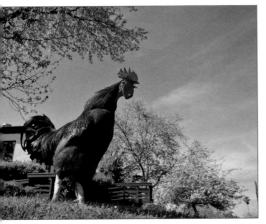

Although noble and invaluable to the small flock owner desiring to increase flock size, the broody and protective trait isn't acceptable when eggs are required daily. The term "to break up a broody" and suggested

LEFT: Roosters live their lives in blissful ignorance of their owner's need to sleep in undisturbed on the weekends.

practices to prevent broodiness (confinement, wire cages left in drafty locations, denial of access to feed and water) are cruel and unnecessary. Broody hens have already gone off their food. Denying access completely will result in liver damage and other complications.

The best practice is to slip on a glove and keep removing the eggs from underneath her. In her own time she will stop trying to fight you for those eggs.

Quieting a Rooster's Crows

The domestic chicken has inherited and kept most of the traits of its wild ancestors. Roosters are a flock's only natural protection. Their crowing, carried on not just in the morning but throughout the entire day, is a territorial warning. You cannot retrain instinct. Accommodations must be made. Although roosters are unnecessary if you don't plan on breeding your hens, many people enjoy their look, their ability to protect the flock, and their wake-up call. Melodious as it may be to you, your neighbors might not be as impressed at 4 A.M. on a Sunday morning.

Outwitting his instinctual nature is an option, but I would suggest that the following methods are neither easy nor entirely effective. Consider giving him away or, if he's young enough, dress him for your freezer.

Crowing is instinctual behavior. This is the rooster's means of protecting and maintaining his flock of hens—his very purpose in life. It can neither be untaught nor discouraged by any means. Surgery is possible, but expensive and inhumane.

To crow, a rooster must stand up tall and crane his neck upward. If you can prevent him from a full stretch, you might be able to quiet his earliest morning crows. This involves catching him every night and bedding him down in a cage that is too short for him to stretch. If you take this route every night while you look for a new home for him, be sure to release him as soon as you awake. It isn't fair to an animal to be awake, instinctively driven to crow, and immobilized.

A more humane short-term option might be to section off a dark corner of the coop and chase him in every night. Your goal is to trick him into believing it is still night until you release him in the morning. If he hears his hens stirring in the morning he may start crowing anyway. At the very least he will be stressed.

Designing Your Small Farm Strategy

After years of switching between various breeds—often raising two classes at a time—I have once again returned to keeping Barred Plymouth Rocks, a dual-purpose breed. My reasons for doing so are based on our family's needs, climate conditions, and available space (both in the coop and in the freezer). Your needs will vary from mine and, as your personal requirements change, over time. To help you determine your best strategy from year to year, here are some of the top considerations before placing your hatchery order.

Meat Birds

- Grow meat birds to whatever size fits your family best. As an example, a family of four that doesn't enjoy leftovers might opt to grow their broilers to a three-pound dressed weight in seven weeks.
- Check your calendar before you order. If you will be butchering the chickens yourself you'll need a few days open for the task seven to nine weeks from the date day-old chicks arrive, or five to seven weeks from the date started chicks arrive. You don't want to overgrow a meat breed when their conversion rates drop. You'll be losing money—potentially losing lives. Past the weight of seven to eight pounds (live weight) feed-to-muscle conversion slows. In my experience, almost all growth over nine pounds (live weight) is stored as fat that just ends up in the garbage bin anyway. Growing to obesity also wreaks havoc on your meat birds' overall health. Obese hybrids have an added sensitivity to heat and are prone to heart attacks.

Egg Layers

- Five or six laying hens at peak production will lay between two and three dozen eggs per week—an ample quantity for the average family of four. Add extra hens to your order and you'll always have an extra dozen to share with (or sell to) friends, family, and neighbors.
- Replace laying hens every two years. Productivity will be dramatically reduced by the third year. Even the hyper-productive Leghorn drops down to one egg every three days at this age.

Timing

- Plan on a spring start and you will move into the fall season with a freezer full of chicken meat and hardy hens laying in the coop.
- Starting with day-olds? You can raise meat birds and laying hens in one partitioned coop. By the time the layers need the space the meat birds will already be in the freezer.
- Dual-purpose cockerels take eighteen to twenty weeks to reach full size; hens take twenty-five to start laying.

Freezer Space

- If your family eats one chicken dinner per week you'll be raising over fifty meat birds throughout the year. Consider the option of raising two sets of twenty-five for fresher poultry throughout the year if your climate permits. Consider owning two smaller freezers and emptying out one halfway through the year to conserve energy.

Ordering

- Some hatcheries will let you specify your order to contain all male (cockerels) or a mix of both sexes. A little more expensive per chick, the males will grow faster and make better use of their food intake. If you grow only cockerels you will have yet one more reason to be committed to your finish date. Cornish-cross cocks—like any other breed—will squabble and crow at maturity. Ensure you get them to the freezer on time and you shouldn't have any problems with coop fights or crowing complaints.

Saving Money Raising Chickens

- All breeds will consume more food during cooler months.
- All breeds need supplementary heat if temperatures drop below 60 degrees Fahrenheit.
- Don't buy or keep a dual-purpose or laying-breed rooster if you don't plan on hatching chicks.
- A laying hen eats twenty-five pounds of grain before she'll lay her first egg. Consider buying started pullets or ready-to-lay hens.
- Running heat lamps, supplementary winter lighting, and coop heaters increases the cost of raising poultry. Minimize coop space for wintered chickens, add insulation, and keep the area draft-free to cut down costs.

The Chicken Coop and Yard

Although you will need to provide a shelter for your chickens, it merely needs to be adequate—adequate protection from extreme temperature and from predators, adequate space to eliminate stress-related illnesses from cramped living quarters, and adequate containment from your personal property and other farm animals' feed.

A shed or a corner of an existing barn will be sufficient. If you must build a coop, the simplest to build is a square building with:

- A slanted roof (rain should run away from the yard)
- Two doors, one for you and one for the chickens
- A ceiling tall enough that you can stand easily inside
- Enough space for the quantity of chickens you desire, plus room to add a few more along the way

> **Building a Stationary Chicken Coop?**
>
> Build it on a slight slope to prevent muddy yards during the rainy seasons.
>
> Build it close enough to a stand of trees to reduce the chilling effect of winter's prevailing winds. At the same time, build it far enough away from the stand of trees to ensure that predators cannot jump from trees to the outside yard.

Have your coop wired for electricity or add in a few solar panels. A heat lamp for new chicks, extra light during the winter for laying hens, and/or a small heater for the coldest nights of the year are practical necessities.

How Much Space?

Recommended space for a full-grown chicken is two to two and a half square feet—quite likely twice as much space as a chicken would receive in a poultry factory. Of the belief that a little more is a lot better, I allot four square feet each. This extra space means less concentration of odor, fewer fights among the flock, a lot less stress for the birds, and more places for you to put your feet when visiting the coop.

Based on my four-square-feet rule, twenty-five chickens of any breed can be housed in a ten-foot by ten-foot (one-hundred-square-foot) space. Add an outdoor run of another four hundred square feet (sixteen square feet each) and your chickens will have ample room to grow, explore, and exercise with few problems.

I apply the same principle when raising meat birds. Old-school farmers and hatcheries state that meat birds don't require as much room nor do they need an outside run. Their theory is that exercising the meat bird wastes feed energy that could be better utilized for building bulk. Although true—that a meat bird's sole purpose is to grow and therefore it does not need outdoor space—fresh air, sunshine, and space enhance their quality of life. When contemplating the blessings these birds give my family, a little extra feed and a little extra space just seems fair.

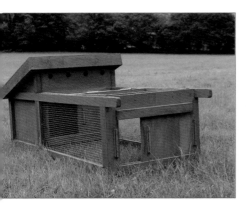

ABOVE: A backyard chicken tractor. Note the handles (for moving) and ventilation holes above the roosting and nesting area on the "top" floor.

Variations of Coops

In the last ten years, one type of chicken housing has been growing in popularity in both urban and country yards. Dubbed the "chicken tractor," these movable coops are made to house four to six chickens comfortably. Tops are hinged to make egg collection, feeding, and water changes a snap. Coop mobility ensures no one area of the yard is compromised and chickens are less likely to develop internal parasitic infestations as a result.

Litter

Spread litter on the floor of your coop and within nesting boxes to absorb smell and feces. Depending on your coop floor and the season, extra litter might also provide insulation. Begin a freshly cleaned coop with four inches of litter, adding an inch of fresh litter when the litter has lost its ability to absorb smell, becomes trampled down, or is noticeably soiled. Completely replace litter during every major cleaning.

Litter can be any soft and absorbent material, such as straw, ground-up corncobs, wood chips and shavings, or shredded paper. Use whichever you can purchase inexpensively and is accessible nearby. Your local feed store might provide leads on sawmills that sell shavings or farmers who sell straw.

Temperature Control

The optimum temperature for chickens is between 45 and 80 degrees Fahrenheit. Extremes on either side may result in less-efficient conversion of feed. Temperature-related troubles include: fewer or smaller eggs, slower-growing meat birds, thin-shelled eggs, frostbitten combs and feet, onset of stress-related sickness, and death.

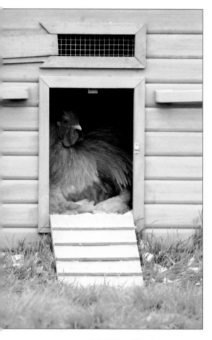

In cooler climates your coop should be completely free of drafts. Add a heat lamp or small heater over the roosting area when temperatures dip below 45 degrees Fahrenheit. Keep in mind that litter could be a fire hazard if kicked onto a floor-based heat source.

Be innovative in conserving electricity when wintering hens. In previous years I have moved laying hens to a smaller shed and have also been known to drop the ceiling on my large coop with securely stapled tarps and Styrofoam insulation above. In northern climates some people will move their hens to a south-facing front or back porch during winter months.

ABOVE: Chickens require shade, extra water, and cross-ventilation during summer. Sliding mesh vents, such as the ones shown in this photo, ensure that air moves freely inside.

When temperatures climb into the high 70s, air will need to move freely and regularly through the coop. Wire-screened windows in the coop allow for cross breezes as do wire mesh gable ends or vents close to floor level (create sliders or board them over for winter).

Coop Cleanliness

Keeping your coop clean serves a dual purpose—your chickens remain healthy and odors are controlled. If you save coop-cleaning chores to once per week, other obligations will almost always take you away. On the other hand, regular maintenance in your twice-daily visits will result in a coop kept nearly as clean as the day your chickens arrived.

Daily chores include checking chickens' dishes, collecting eggs (if raising layers), and opening or closing yard access. Take just a few minutes, every now and then, to add new litter, sweep dust off rafters and walls, change nesting materials, or remove wet litter from the base of watering stations. You'll now have your weekends free to enjoy your chickens from the back porch with your feet up.

A few minutes here and there, a complete litter change every four to eight weeks (depending on odor), and a clean-and-disinfect session once to twice per year is all that is required to have happy chickens with a coop you'll be proud to show off.

Coop Equipment

Equipment to outfit your chicken coop is minimal. You'll need food and water containers and, if raising laying hens, perches and nesting boxes.

Roosters and hens are instinctively territorial, and feeding stations are within the dominion of territory. Although it may seem excessive, provide two watering and feeding stations per twenty-five chickens. The extra feeders and founts are a preventative measure that ensures every bird has access to food and water without stress. This measure of prevention turns to necessity should you introduce new birds to an existing flock or if you own more than one rooster in a large flock.

Founts

Chickens need access to water at all times and will consume one to two cups of water per day each.

Daily consumption varies per bird and across the seasons. A laying hen can drink twice as much as a meat bird of equal size.

During hot summer days your chickens can drink up to twice as much water as usual to keep their body temperature manageable. I like to add an extra fount in a shady spot of their yard to ensure they have quick and easy access to water at all times. In the winter an electric or solar powered de-icer saves you six trips to the coop to ensure your hens stay hydrated.

An inexpensive galvanized fount can last you many years. They are easy to handle, are quickly disinfected with a mild bleach solution, and should they ever crack, a quick bead of epoxy repairs them.

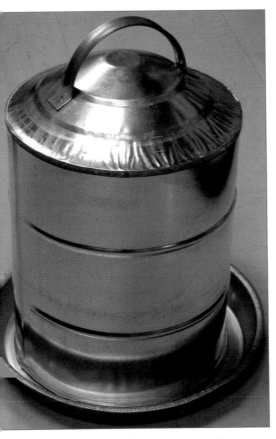

ABOVE: Galvanized watering founts are priced to fit your budget and last for many years.

If you keep founts elevated you'll prevent waste from collecting in the trough area and rust from ruining the base.

I've never been fond of plastic as a long-term solution, but the small plastic founts are perfect when you need to quarantine a hen or when you are starting young chicks. Keep larger plastic founts out of direct sunlight and do not use if a chance of freezing exists. Plastic founts are prone to crack in extremes and may leach toxins into the water if not made of BPA-free plastic.

Dirty watering stations are a breeding ground for bacteria. Changing the water daily and sanitizing the fount weekly are as important as having an ample supply. Chickens are notorious for drinking with food in their mouths and kicking litter into the trough. Alleviate both problems by moving founts away from feeders and raising them off the floor to the chickens' chest level.

Feeders

As with water, chickens need to eat all day long to stay healthy and remain free of stress.

The rule of thumb is one five-gallon feeder for every twenty-five chickens plus one extra for every rooster in the coop. Even if you don't have two roosters, keep two feeders in operation to ensure chickens lower in the pecking order don't go hungry.

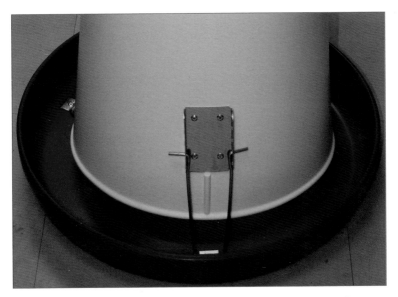

ABOVE: The base of this feeder has a curved side and a rolled rim, lessening the amount of food wasted by chickens billing out their feed.

Chickens have no respect for household economics and are notorious for picking through feed for choice bits, dumping out and wasting a huge amount of feed. If you adjust the height of the feed basin to match their chest level and purchase a feeder with a rim that rolls inward, you can prevent the costly habit known as billing out. Hanging feeders allow you to make height adjustments as your chickens grow.

Another wasteful but preventable habit is when chickens roost upon the feeder top and soil the feed within. Hanging feeders deter them, but if they persist, add more roosting space in your coop and cut an upturned plastic bucket for a custom-fit cover.

Supplement Feeders

All chickens store and use grit in their gizzards to grind up food for digestion. Although chickens with outside access will obtain some grit naturally, they aren't likely to find all they need in a small yard. Ask your feed store if grit is included in your feed, and if not, add a small bag and a supplement feeder to your order.

Laying hens require calcium in their diets to form eggshells and keep their production cycles strong. Adequate calcium is already added to most laying ration. If your hens have access to a yard they'll also obtain calcium from eating hard-shelled insects. If you sense that your hens aren't receiving enough calcium in their diets, you can purchase it separately and provide it, free-choice, in a small feeder. As with granite grit, your chickens will not eat more than they need.

Special Considerations for Laying Hens

Perches

Instinctively, laying hens roost at night. If you don't provide a perch for them they will do their level best to rest (and mess on) their nesting boxes, food and water containers, feed sacks, ceiling rafters, or anything else they can reach. Furthermore, if perches aren't supplied, hens will fight for the best spot, feel overcrowded, and put themselves in danger (ascending and descending from ceiling rafters, for instance).

Perches should be made of one- to two-inch wood with slightly rounded edges. Allow twelve inches of roosting space per hen and keep perches a minimum of eighteen inches from the wall. Droppings are at their worst under roosting space. Elongated boot trays or a mechanic's plastic oil pan makes frequent cleanups a cinch.

Note: Meat birds might play and exercise on perches early in their lives, but you should discontinue access by the time they are five weeks of age because they become large and clumsy. If you decide to allow low perches for meat birds (six inches off the floor only), ensure they have at least two feet of space between wall and perch and eighteen to twenty inches of perch each.

Nesting Boxes

Instinctively a chicken knows to lay eggs in a nesting box. You don't need to teach her to do so; you simply need to provide an adequate box.

If you don't provide a nest, the hens will leave their eggs on the floor. Within minutes the eggs become soiled, cracked, pecked at, and potentially eaten by the others. A minor loss today becomes a serious loss in the future. Egg-eating quickly turns into a coop-wide bad habit that cannot be untaught.

There are a variety of nest styles to choose from. Hanging nests, free-standing dark nests, and even sturdy wood crates raised just a few inches off the floor. Your hens won't be picky but they might have a favorite out of the ones you provide.

You can be creative with nests you make or provide; just be sure they allow for your easy access. A friend once built a partial wall of nests that was accessed by one large hinged door of round holes. She had the coolest coop for miles but collecting eggs in the top row of nests—where you couldn't easily see what you were collecting—wasn't fun. Sometimes what she'd pull out was just a round ball of poop. Ugh.

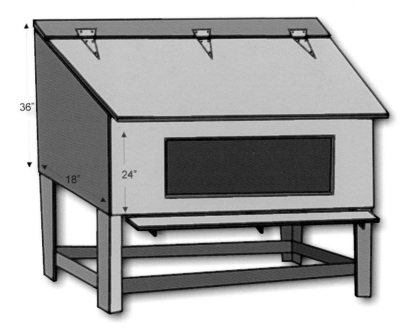

ABOVE: The dark nest is a lumber-saving, age-old design that makes egg collection and cleaning easy.

Over the years I've discovered a passion for the dark nest. Built of plywood and constructed in just a few hours, the dark nest can be used by multiple hens without squabbling or rivalry. Each hen requires only twelve inches of nest within so you'll save on space and material if you need to build nesting boxes anyway. Include a perch on the front and your hens won't be apprehensive upon entering the dark nest.

Dimensions are not specific as the dark nest can be custom fit to your coop space. The slanted and hinged roof prevents hens from roosting above and allows easy access for egg collection. Rest the finished box on concrete blocks or build it with posts so it is two or more feet off the floor. Adjust the elevation to save your back, as you'll be stooping over every morning to collect eggs.

If you plan on building individual nesting boxes, here are some general guidelines:

- A size of fourteen inches square works for all sizes of laying hens.
- A lip on the front keeps eggs and nesting material safely inside.
- A height of two feet from the floor might be easiest for the hens, but not so easy on your back. Most hens will use nesting boxes three to four feet off the ground as long as they have the means and the space to ascend and descend without stress.
- A perch in front alleviates stress for hens wanting in and hens already settled inside.
- Three to four inches of litter or nesting material, changed regularly, keeps the area clean and odor free.

Lighting

Laying hens require thirteen to fourteen hours of light per day for optimum health and production. In North America this is only a problem during the shortest winter days.

Although you may be tempted to move your hens to a covered and sunny porch during winter, allow me to remind you of the dust they can create in just a few days. You'll love your hens more if you leave them where they are, insulate and heat your coop, and add artificial light for the winter months. I've found the best results using one standard incandescent bulb and one full-spectrum grow light from the gardening section.

The Chicken Yard

Your chickens will be happiest and healthiest when given outdoor room to roam. They will roll in soil, forage for bugs, pull up roots, ingest sprouts, and enjoy the natural benefits of the sun. If you can provide them a safe place to enjoy acting like chickens and are thrilled to do so, you will be equally distressed to find that within a month's time their yard is a packed-dirt and barren wasteland.

Some say there is no way around it, that chickens will annihilate any yard you give them in short order. I say there is an alternative.

If you build a coop in the center of a divided chicken yard or build a large yard around your coop, you can rotate access to four quadrants while keeping each area viable. This is similar to the rotational-grazing method that manages larger livestock pastures. Concerning chickens, however, rotational grazing is much easier to implement. Four chicken doors within the coop allow you to dictate on a day-by-day basis which quadrant of the yard they will access.

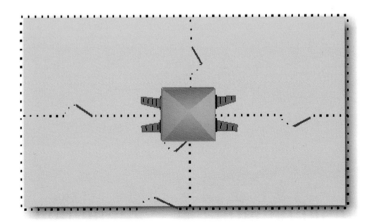

ABOVE: Quad yard for chickens. More gates to build than a standard yard, but so much nicer for chickens that can't wander about freely.

The most trouble-free birds are those who have at least four times the fenced space out of doors that they have indoors.

My first 10- by 12-foot coop (120 square feet), which comfortably housed two dozen large laying hens, had a 3,000-square-foot yard sectioned into quarters (each quarter being 25 by 30 feet or 750 square feet). Considered overkill by old-school farming standards, this arrangement kept the hens happy and I felt satisfied in the way I provided for them.

Fencing

Chickens are absolutely incapable of defending themselves and every potential predator knows it. Foxes, hawks, wolves, weasels, and raccoons will jump at any opportunity to take one or more of your flock. The list of potential predators doesn't stop at wildlife. Mild-mannered family pets have also been known to annihilate an entire flock of chickens in less than an hour.

You may be one of the fortunate few who can free-range hens without a loss for years. It was once possible on my farm, too, but in the last five years a large population of coyotes and foxes has moved in. Although I dislike fencing the chickens in, I appease the desire to let them roam free just a few times each year now.

A standard chicken yard fence is four feet high with posts spaced six to eight feet apart. Posts are buried two feet into the soil and, along with corner supports, are located within the perimeter of the fence. Wily and nimble predators can and will climb fence supports if they're left on the outsides of the corners.

Chicken wire is inexpensive and easy to handle, but the strongest fence is built of a medium-gauge yard and garden wire. With one-inch square holes in the bottom quarter and larger holes on top, this fencing material can keep chicks as young as a month old on the inside and most predators out.

If weasels and raccoons are a nuisance in your area, consider attaching sturdy wire to the underside of the coop.

Perhaps the best defense against predators is to be mindful of the signs they leave from one night to the next. Should you notice a gnawed board, wire that has been pulled away from the post, or roofing material pulled off the coop, take immediate action. Many predators have been known to return night after night until they gain access. Never put off an issue of safety until tomorrow. Tomorrow may never come for your chickens.

Your family dog is also a great defense, but only as a deterrent. While some farmers might tie their dogs near the coop to sound an alarm, this strategy can have dire consequences for the dog should a pack of wolves or a lone cougar wander through.

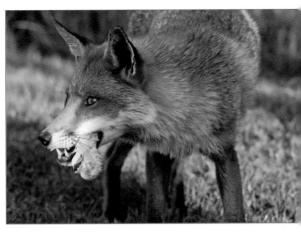

ABOVE: In broad daylight with the farmer nearby, this bold fox takes a chicken's life and then stands in open terrain enjoying his lunch.

If you have persistent problems with a particular animal, discuss the situation with other locals who keep chickens. Local wildlife authorities might also have solutions or insight into the problem.

An Afternoon Out for the Girls

Should you decide to let your hens out a few times a year to wander in your gardens and enjoy a little extra space, you'll want to keep close watch. I only open the gate when I know I'll be spending the next few hours outside, and I ensure each one follows me into the yard, never leaving my line of sight. After the incident with a very bold coyote just three feet away, I also take my rifle.

I have yet to lose a hen doing so, but only because:

- We have cleared acreage. If a predator is stalking he'd be hard-pressed to sneak up on us.
- A hen will seldom roam from the safety of the flock or within a safe running distance of her coop. Should any of them leave the flock they most often end up at my feet.

· I spend a lot of time with my layers. If I need to get them back into their coop early I just call them in. (There's nothing magical to this—I simply conditioned them to the call of scratch grain—you can do it too!)

Where to Buy Chickens

Chicks can be purchased at country auctions, from a local farmer, by mail order, or direct from a reputable hatchery.

My best birds have consistently arrived from a hatchery. Although I've purchased some hens and a few roosters at auction and privately, too much is at stake to risk a chance on parasitic infestation and disease. An entire coop can get sick overnight and all will be lost for the sake of one small purchase.

In twelve years I have heard a hundred or more similar tales of woe from my readers on GoodByeCityLife.com. Here are just a few ways that purchasing chicks can go wrong.

You Can't Always Trust a Seller. One couple purchased three day-old pullets at a farmer's market. After raising and caring for the chicks for nearly four months, two of their pullets grew to be cockerels, but they seemed to be getting along with each other. Returning home from work one afternoon they discovered the smaller rooster lying nearly dead on the driveway and the larger one delivering some fierce final blows.

Mail-Order Chicks Arrive Dead. A young woman, living remotely and on a quest for self-sustained living, ordered thirty chicks by mail order. Arriving at the courier pickup location on time and excited, she found that the box was full of dead chicks.

Accounts from other readers have cited boxes of chicks that are travel-weary and stressed to the point of sickness.

Receiving chicks by mail order has lost the reliable reputation it once held. The best hatcheries will guarantee live delivery, but that merely equates to a credit of replacement chicks if yours arrive dead. Day-old chicks are shipped by plane (in the cargo bay), by regular postal trucks, or through courier services. Although a newly hatched chick is capable of surviving without food or water for twenty-four hours, it is not capable of thriving in impossible temperatures or managing the stress of being consistently jostled about. A delivery service is not concerned about stress, temperature, or whether live cargo arrives alive or not—they receive the same payment either way.

One New Hen Sickens an Entire Flock. I've done this myself. At a livestock auction I met a knowledgeable and friendly seller with a hen I just had to have. I inspected her for lice, leg mites, and overall health, and she seemed perfectly sound. During quarantine the hen became listless and weak and eventually died. Had I released her into the general population I might have lost my entire flock.

The lesson here is no matter how experienced any of us think we might be about raising chickens, or how trustworthy we believe a seller to be, we can always be taken by surprise. Make your purchase from a recommended and local hatchery, no matter how small your order, and arrange to pick up your order personally and directly.

Your feed store might offer a service of pre-ordering and accepting delivery for annual chick orders. The hatchery delivers organized boxes to the feed store and the chicks inside are quickly inspected before you pick them up. This minimizes delivery stress, improper handling, and time in transit.

Ordering and Caring for Chickens

Chickens from commercial growers are sold as day-olds, started (two to four weeks old), and ready to lay. You can further specify whether you'd like cockerels, pullets, or straight-run chicks.

Straight-run orders are filled as the chicks hatch and are therefore cheaper. When raising meat birds, a straight-run order will give you wider variety in finished size. When ordering dual-purpose breeds as straight-run chicks, you'll have the best of both worlds—roosters to cull for the freezer and hens to keep for laying.

Day-Old Chicks

Day-old chicks cost about two-thirds less than started birds. They are often pulled dry from the incubator, vaccinated for Marek's disease, and popped into the box for delivery.

Once home, you will need a heat lamp to keep the chicks warm for a few weeks. One 250-watt infrared lamp will keep fifty to a hundred chicks warm, but keep two in case one should fail. A hanging heat lamp placed eighteen to twenty-four inches from the floor allows you to make adjustments from day to night and as chicks grow.

There are two ways to ensure the temperature is perfect for young chicks. The first is to take a temperature reading of 90 to 92 degrees Fahrenheit, two inches off the floor. The second is by observing the chicks' behavior. Chicks that are too cold will pile on top of each other under the lamp and chirp. If they are too warm they'll wander away from the lamp or lie down with wings spread and panting if they can't get far enough away. A sign of correct heating is when chicks are freely wandering within the perimeter of the lamp and occasionally returning to bask in some

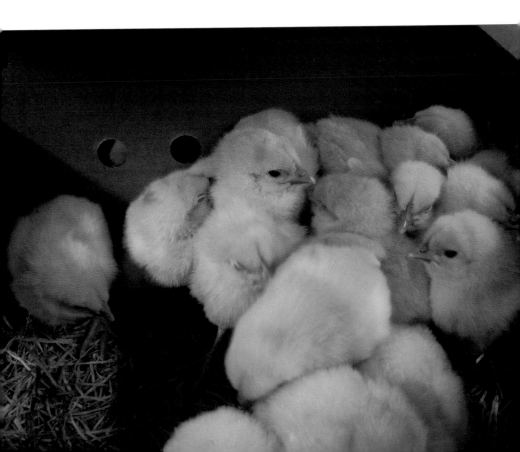

extra warmth. Feed and water dishes should rest just outside of the lamp's radius.

If chicks will be kept in an area where pets might enter, or that might be drafty, start your chicks in a solid-wall brooding box that is vented above. Brooding boxes can be as simple as a sturdy cardboard box or as elaborate as a fine mesh kennel protected on all sides. If chicks are going directly into a new coop where no other animal can get at them, you can skip the brooder—they are not likely to leave the immediate vicinity of the heat source or the safety of their brood mates.

Keep your chicks' area clean and dry with a constant supply of fresh water and feed. A base of newspaper with paper toweling on top is absorbent, can be easily changed, and will prevent slippery mishaps. Wood shavings or sawdust are not recommended as litter for young chicks. Chicks will ingest the shavings and end up with swollen, impacted crops that will eventually kill them.

Chicks will have to be taught how and where to drink. Dip a few chicks' beaks into lukewarm water from a small fount (provide one fount for every fifty chicks) and the others should catch on. Don't be shy about being overprotective and dipping every beak—I do it!

After the first week and every week thereafter, adjust the height of the fount to the chicks' chest level to keep kicked litter out of the basin. Make similar adjustments for feeders.

As your chicks grow they will spend less time under the lamp. Make adjustments for their age, the temperature of the room they're in, or by time of day. If I'm starting chicks in a cool spring I'll raise the heat lamp every week by an inch (thereby decreasing temperature by 5 degrees) and eventually turn the light off for daylight hours. They are fine as long as they aren't chirping loudly and huddling. By six weeks they should be acclimatized, but the exact time to remove it altogether is dependent on coop temperature

LEFT: Meat birds from the hatchery, directly to you. Freshly hatched chicks are vaccinated, then packed into a box and shipped to the consumer. The chickens in the back of this box are huddling for warmth but are not stressed at the end of their journey.

(no lower than 65 degrees Fahrenheit). Close observation of their behavior without the lamp is the best cue.

Started Chicks and Ready-to-Lay Pullets

Started chicks are a nice option for the new farmer. Arriving between two and four weeks of age, vaccinated for Marek's, and fed a medicated feed to kick-start immunity to coccidiosis, your chickens arrive young enough to bond with, but more established than a day-old.

A four-week-old chick is capable of dealing with low nightly temperatures of 75 degrees Fahrenheit. If seasonal temperatures in your region drop below 75 degrees, add a heat lamp (instructions above in the Day-Old Chicks section) until you're sure it is no longer required.

Ready-to-lay pullets (sold at sixteen to twenty weeks of age) may have just started laying eggs or will begin within the next few weeks. I like to call them "instant egg layers in a box"—just add coop, feed, and water.

It is common hatchery practice to leave the lights on for twelve hours a day when raising pullets, and to suggest that you increase their day's light by one extra hour over the course of a week, for the next four weeks—to a maximum of sixteen hours per day. I usually purchase hens in the summer months and let Mother Nature manage the light until winter arrives.

Saving Money on Your Chick Order

Chickens are sold by the hatcheries on a sliding scale. The larger number of birds you purchase, the lower price per bird you'll pay. If you can double up your order with one or more friends you can save as much as $1 per chick.

If you're ordering laying hens, you can pay just a few dollars more per hen and get ready-to-lay pullets, which will save you the cost of twenty-five pounds of feed per hen and the need for heat lamps.

If your heart isn't set on a particular breed, check your hatchery for special deals on overruns and mixed lots. You can often save 50 percent per order through hatchery specials.

Caring for and Feeding Chickens

Commercial feeds are available to suit each changing need of your flock—starting, growing, maintenance, and finishing mixtures—in a choice of three consistencies: mash, crumbles, or pellets. For starting chicks I use crumbles for the first eight weeks, then switch over to pellets for the remainder. Mash has consistently been a dusty waste in my coop.

A few weeks before your hens are expected to begin laying (eighteen weeks for laying breeds, twenty-two weeks for dual-purpose breeds), start changing their feed over to a layer's pellet a little at a time at first until they are on straight laying ration.

If you've purchased straight-run, dual-purpose chicks, this twenty-two-week mark is also a good time to move out the cockerels. Grow them a little longer on grower ration or dress them for the freezer as your time permits.

The meat breeds can be switched over to grower ration by four weeks of age. You will not need to switch their feed again unless you choose to give them a finishing ration in the final weeks.

Another popular feed, but one to stay away from, is scratch grain. Deceptive in appearance, scratch grain looks like it might be the most natural feed for your chickens. Ounce per ounce it is also the cheapest. Scratch grain lacks in required protein and calcium for layers and is not suitable for fast-growing meat breed crosses. Use scratch grain as a treat or training aid only.

Poor-quality feed with nutrient deficiencies creates internal imbalances. Dietary deficiency is the most common culprit for poor egg production or slow-growing meat birds.

How Much Chicken Feed to Buy

Twenty-five two-week-old meat breed chicks eat at least twenty-five pounds of feed per week.

Twenty-five four-week-old meat breed chicks eat at least fifty pounds of feed per week.

Twenty-five eight-week-old meat breed chicks eat well over a hundred pounds of feed per week, now at their prime of converting feed to muscle.

Twenty-five laying chicks (up to twenty weeks of age) will eat approximately twenty-five pounds of feed per week. (Obviously less in the beginning and more towards maturity.)

Twenty-five mature laying hens eat fifty pounds of feed per week.

Save on Feed Costs

Almost 60 percent of the cost of keeping chickens is spent on feed. Although your chickens will show you their own style of wasting feed, other factors are within your control. The following are my top five tips for saving money on feed costs.

- In an effort to save money while raising your own food, the question comes to mind: "Why feed a rooster?"
- At the feed store, when given the choice between mash, pellets, or crumbles for birds over eight weeks old, choose pellets. Less feed will be wasted.
- Know how much feed you'll need for three weeks at a time and save gas running to the feed store every week. Keep feed bags dry and out of direct sun to protect against rot and staleness, respectively. Rodents such as chipmunks, mice, and rats can chew their way through the bottom of any feed bag or plastic tub and consume or contaminate the entire lot. Keep feed in the bag within a clean galvanized trash bin.
- Feed your chickens as much vegetable scrap from the kitchen and clippings from the garden as possible. The more you feed them from your farm and table, the less

commercial feed you'll pay for. A few exceptions are potato peelings (which are not digestible) and pungent produce such as garlic and onions (which taint the taste of meat and eggs). Most other fruits and vegetables will surely be consumed and enjoyed by your flock. You can help put calcium back into a chicken's digestion by feeding empty eggshells to them. Just be sure to grind them up well past recognition before delegating them back to the coop.

· Plan on getting meat birds to the freezer before or as soon as possible after their ninth week. Their feed-to-meat conversion ratio begins to decline at this age.

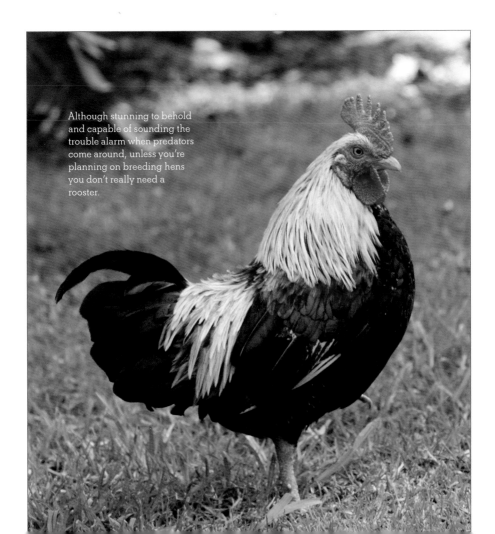

Although stunning to behold and capable of sounding the trouble alarm when predators come around, unless you're planning on breeding hens you don't really need a rooster.

Maintain Good Health in Your Flock

Ninety percent of success in raising chickens can be found in these two words: obtain and maintain. When chickens arrive on your land healthy, it doesn't take much to maintain that state. Clean living conditions, lack of stress, and an adequate supply of clean water are the top three preventative measures against sickness.

Vaccinations are another consideration to ensuring your chickens stay healthy. As some bacterial viruses and diseases are localized, ask a veterinarian in your area if any special vaccinations are required.

Prevent disease, virus, and infection being unknowingly introduced to your coop:

- Rodents and wild birds are notorious for spreading disease as they travel from coop to coop. Manage rodent population with traps or by ensuring they can't get at feed and grain. Without easy access to food, rodents won't stick around. Wild birds can be kept out of the chicken yard by adding aviary netting across the top of your yard fence.
- Some chickens are only carriers of a disease and show no signs of illness. Only purchase chickens to add to a flock from a hatchery and quarantine every new chicken for at least a week before introducing it to existing flocks.
- Just as introducing new chickens to a coop can cause the spread of a disease, so might the soles of your shoes carry in sickness if you've visited another coop. Before you head off to your own chores, clean and sanitize your shoes after spending time at another coop.

Catching illness before it becomes a deadly outbreak isn't easy. Your senses have to be fully present for each chicken in the coop, every time you enter the coop. Once familiar with your chickens, you'll pick up on changes that could be a signal of sickness. Loss of weight or lack of growth in a young bird, consistent drooping heads or hunched appearances, change in comb color or size, dripping noses or eyes, rattling chests, and changes in stool droppings are but a few signs of various illnesses.

Symptoms can be confusing. As an example, loose stools may be attributed to coccidiosis, and decreased laying or weight loss might be a sign of worm infestation, but coupled with other changes these symptoms might signal something worse.

If you notice illness in just one chicken, immediately quarantine it. If all your chickens appear sick, call a veterinarian for further instruction.

It is a fact of life and of raising chickens that not all diseases can be noted and cured in time. In most cases, by the time you notice that a chicken is sick, it is already too late. Even if you could cure the disease and nurse your hen back to health, she might remain a carrier and pass the disease on to others.

Parasitic Infestations

Of the two—internal and external—the most unnerving parasites are external. Unchecked lice and mites quickly turn into a coop infestation. They can arrive on your chickens, can live in your coop from one batch of chickens to the next, and if left untreated, can drag your chickens to death's door.

Lice and mites spread quickly from one bird to another. You'll only need to check one or two birds to know if you need to take immediate action. Visit the coop after dark with a friend and a flashlight. Don't startle sleeping chickens on the roost by waving the light in their faces, just calmly collect one off the roost and shine the flashlight to the base of the feathers by the head, vent, and under the wings.

Lice will leave signs of eggs that look like tiny rice grains. They will also leave scabs on your bird's skin where they've bitten and chewed.

Mites come in two forms—body mites and leg mites.

There will be no mistaking body mites under the flashlight's beam. They look like tiny red spiders crawling on your chicken's skin.

Raised scales on a chicken's legs are a sign of leg mites. Leg mites are discouraged, controlled, and smothered by coating perches and the legs of chickens with daily applications of vegetable oil or petroleum jelly for seven to ten days.

Body mites and lice require a thorough coop cleanout, poultry-safe insecticidal powder, and diligence to the directions on the label.

Coccidiosis

Coccidiosis is an intestinal disease that can weaken and kill untreated chicks. Most adult chickens have an immunity to the organism that causes it, but can still suffer from the disease. You will instantly recognize the spread of this illness by loose droppings throughout the coop. Medication can be readily purchased at any feed supply store.

Starter feed for chicks often contains Amprolium, a medication developed to control intestinal coccidia while allowing chickens time to build up a natural immunity. Ask at the feed store if Amprolium is present in your feed, and then make a personal decision about the value of pre-medicating poultry that is not sick.

Marek's Disease

Marek's disease is a cancer-causing viral infection. The disease is spread via feather dander and inhalation. Most hatcheries automatically vaccinate for Marek's within the first few hours of hatching.

The Joy of Eggs

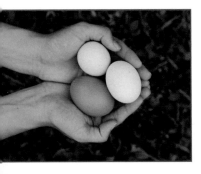

Crack a farm-fresh egg into your frying pan and you'll find a firm white with a deep-orange and substantial yolk. These eggs look and cook a little differently than the grocer's version. Yolks are darker, whites are firmer, and the air sac within is most certainly smaller. Higher density and less air space within the shell makes these eggs economical as well. Fewer farm-fresh eggs are required for large batch baking, and the whites create more volume when whipped.

As for the grocer's version of an egg, the time to market has some bearing on the lack of quality and taste, as most eggs are already a week old by the time they hit your shopping cart. However, a hen's diet and living conditions are the two main contributors affecting the taste and density of any egg—farm-fresh or commercial.

Years ago I was surprised to learn that farm-fresh eggs can be as dull as the commercial egg. For years my in-laws raised cooped-up Leghorns that were never allowed to forage on the land, never given garden or table scraps, and never enjoyed the wonders of direct sunlight. Take note: if you don't take the route of reproducing an egg factory in your own coop, you won't run the risk of having unspectacular eggs.

Give your layers a yard of sunshine, clean and spacious living conditions, fresh water at all times, and a varied diet. You'll be well rewarded for your efforts.

Freshness Tests

As eggs sit in storage (whether destined for the grocery store or awaiting use in your own refrigerator), they lose moisture through the shell. This evaporation creates an air bubble noticeable only when you hard boil the egg or hold it to a light source. If you're uncertain how old an egg is, check the bubble. Fresh eggs have virtually no hollow within the shell.

You can also float an egg to see if it is fresh. Fresh eggs sink in a bowl of water. An egg that stands upright is only a few days old. Older eggs float and aren't fit for consumption.

Cleaning and Storing Eggs

Freshly collected eggs have an invisible layer of protection upon them called a bloom. The bloom keeps moisture in and surrounding air out. If you scrub off the bloom before storage you compromise the egg's natural ability to stay fresh. A quick rinse in water slightly warmer than the egg maintains the integrity of bloom during storage.

Keep your eggs in the vegetable tray of your refrigerator—even if space is tight. Specialty shelves on the fridge door are not actually suitable for egg storage. Inconsistent temperatures and frequent jumbling about each time the door is opened will age eggs well before their time. Eggs gathered fresh and stored in a crisper easily stay fresh for a month.

There will be times when you have an abundance of eggs and no time to use them all. You can freeze them (out of the shell) for future baking with just a shake of the salt shaker per half dozen. I beat them in lots of four and six, as those are the quantities most often called for in the recipes I use. Freeze them in small glass bowls with tight-fitting lids or BPA-free freezer bags.

A Closer Look at Farm-Raised Eggs

Let's clear this up once and for all: The color of an egg's shell does not determine nutritional quality.

The belief that a brown egg is higher in nutritional value than a white egg is a throwback from past generations. For the last thirty years, most laying hens raised commercially were white egg breeds. On the flip side, most layers raised on the farm were dual-purpose breeds, most of which lay brown eggs. Since we already know that farm-raised eggs are of higher nutritional value, you can see where the confusion began. Imagine the misconceptions that will arise once the Araucana and Ameraucana's eggs gain in popularity! These eggs have shells in various shades of blue, green, and olive.

Yolk color suffers from similar misconceptions. It is not the freshness of the egg that has the greatest impact on yolk color, but the diet of the hen that laid it. Free-range and partial-range hens' eggs will have a dark golden to orange yolk. It is the adequate supply of fresh greens in the diet that creates the coveted hue. If your hens don't get out much or if you find your eggs to be dull in winter months, you can supplement their lay ration with kitchen scraps of broccoli, green beans, and lettuce.

On occasion you might find colored spots within an egg. The spots within unfertilized eggs are completely natural and harmless, although not necessarily desirable. The cause is the tiny blood vessels within the hen during formation of the egg. It will not harm you to eat it or the egg it appeared in, but you might prefer to remove it before cooking. The common misconception is that this is a sign of embryonic development. Most laying hens have never seen a rooster.

DID YOU KNOW?

You need to add two minutes to your cooking time when boiling farm-fresh eggs.

Soft-boiled store-bought eggs = Three minutes
Soft-boiled farm-fresh eggs = Five minutes
Hard-boiled store-bought eggs = Ten minutes
Hard-boiled farm-fresh eggs = Twelve minutes

How to Hard-Boil Fresh Eggs

Try this the next time you need to make a plate of devilled eggs for tomorrow's community dinner using the eggs you collected just this morning.

After hard-boiling fresh eggs from the barn, run cold tap water over the pot of eggs for one minute. Allow the eggs to rest in cold water for another four minutes. Break each shell by applying slight pressure while rolling the egg on the counter. Peel the eggs under water. The result? A perfectly peeled, fresh hard-boiled egg without the telling lack-of-freshness gap seen in aged eggs.

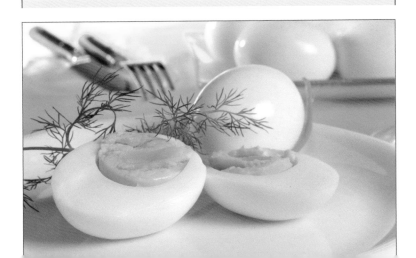

Butchering

The day will come when, either individually or as a lot, your chickens are ready for the butcher. You can take on the task yourself—farm wives and children have been doing it for centuries—as long as you don't intend to sell the chicken to others. Each chicken will take about twenty minutes to prepare for the freezer.

If you're pressed for time, have more than twenty chickens to butcher, or don't have the stomach for the task or volunteer assistants, there are other reasonably priced options for the backyard chicken farmer.

Poultry Processing Services

Scattered throughout North America, you'll find people charging just a few dollars a bird to come to your property and take your chickens from coop to freezer for you. They arrive at your door with a trailer full of equipment and supplies. Asking for nothing more than directions to the barn and the closest hookup for a hose, they set to work and a few hours later return with bags upon bags of perfectly plucked and dressed chickens.

If they don't mind you helping and you don't slow them down, spending a few hours with this group is an education in itself. You will quickly learn the most efficient and health-safe methods to move a chicken from coop to plastic bag.

Often run as a cash-only seasonal business, the service may not be as professional as you'd like. The owner may not be government-certified, so you will need to assess your comfort level with having this group handle food that will one day be on your dinner table. You are also unlikely to find these people in the yellow pages. Ask people in your area also raising chickens for referrals and contact numbers.

The alternative to the on-site butcher is a professional facility that specializes in homegrown poultry. You deliver live chickens to the facility, and then return the next day for pickup. Unlike the on-site option, you need to have enough chickens to make it worth two trips to the facility. These specialists are government-inspected and licensed, and are found in the yellow pages. If you can't locate one, ask for referrals from feed store staff.

Do It Yourself

If you've never butchered poultry, the best preparation is to spend a day with an experienced person. Offer to pay an old-timer or a farm wife in cash, or with a return of time, for a half day of work processing poultry for the freezer. No finer instruction exists than to learn hands-on with experience by your side.

The instructions below are not intended as a complete education in butchering chickens, but merely a guideline of the process.

The Day Before

Feed given twenty-four to thirty hours previous will be found sitting in the chicken's crop, wasted. Time the chickens' last meal so that you are neither wasting feed nor adding unnecessary cleaning chores to the task.

Setting Up

This is an outside, messy task. Wear comfortable chore clothes. You'll need a work table, an axe, a large pot or bin of hot water, sharp knives, poultry shears, a small set of pliers, rubber gloves, garbage bags, easy access to running water, and if possible a screened tent or garden gazebo to work under. Flies and wasps will be exceptionally annoying.

Inside the house you'll need a sanitized sink or basin full of cold salted water. You'll also need to have large plastic freezer bags on hand.

If you're planning on butchering more than four chickens, having some company (even if just a radio playing) keeps monotony at bay.

Order of the Day

The order to be performed is:

- Catch and kill the chicken
- Allow it to bleed out
- Scald, pluck, and gut

- Soak to chill
- Bag for the fridge or freezer

If you've trained them, catching the first few chickens is easy. After three you'll have no choice but to corner each, one by one. Chickens sense that today is different than all other days. They are hungry, members of their flock are being carted out, a commotion can be heard outside, and the smell of trouble is in the air.

An Honorable Death

Knowing that you've *intentionally* raised to *eventually* kill can be unsettling the first time. It becomes less unnerving every year but it is never without emotion. Having a weak spot for animals by nature, I've somehow grown to adopt the farmer's creed: "If you raise it to eat it, you had better be man enough to kill it."
In the end I count it honorable to perform this task myself whenever possible rather than have a stranger attend to it. I literally thank each chicken I carry to the chopping block. Whoever should perform the task, it should be carried out calmly and swiftly. Stress and suffering does nothing for the taste and texture of meat, nor does it honor the life that feeds you.

There must be fifty ways to kill a chicken. The workers at the slaughterhouse hang them by their feet on a moving rack, dip their heads into an electrified bath, and then slit their throats as they pass by. The traveling poultry trailer places chickens upside down in a killing cone, stretches their necks out, cuts their throats, and lets them bleed out from the cone. Small growers also use cones and pierce the chicken's brain through the back of the mouth with a sharp pick or knife.

Killing cones are popular tools of choice. They are inexpensive at the feed supply store, or you can make your own. A round plastic two- or three-gallon jug with the spout and the base cut off works fine. Chickens can hang in the cone until they have fully bled out, containing the mess to one area.

It has been said that if you hold a chicken upside down for a minute it will go to sleep. This has never worked for me because I'm not one to stand the sound of a scared bird. Instead I remove each chicken from the coop and calm it. With one hand on both feet and the chicken's chest laid on the chopping block, I swing the axe. Immediately lifting and holding my chicken away from my body, I allow it to flap unrestricted for about a minute to bleed out. The belief is that flapping assists in pumping the blood out of the body.

Do be careful either to let wings flap without restriction or not at all. Knocks and bumps will bruise the meat of the bird.

A Quick Scald

Once bled out and with head fully removed, hold the chicken by the feet and dip into 140-degrees-Fahrenheit water repeatedly for forty-five to sixty seconds. Dipping is an art in itself—dip longer if water is not quite hot enough, shorter for water hotter than the recommended temperature. The outcome will be loosened feathers without burned skin underneath. Some chickens take a little longer, some a little less.

As soon as you remove the chicken from the water, lay it on the work table and start plucking. Pull feathers, by the handful, in the direction they were growing. This only takes a few minutes per bird if you're working alone. Cut off the feet at the joint, then rinse off the chicken and your work surface with cold running water.

A Cleaning Out

Laying the chicken back onto the work surface, remove the tail and the pointed oil gland at the base of the tail. Ensure that all the yellow substance inside the gland is removed. Using poultry shears or a boning knife, remove the neck and pull the crop and windpipe out from the cavity you've just created.

Splitting a young chicken up the back with poultry shears makes the remainder of the cleaning out process easy and educational for an inexperienced butcher. It affords the observation of the inner workings of a chicken before you ever decide to reach blindly inside to remove entrails.

Whether splitting or processing as a whole bird, take care not to pierce the green bile sac of the liver. It will taint and ruin any meat it touches.

To butcher a chicken whole, make a shallow, somewhat keyhole-shaped incision from the base of the rib cage nearly to the vent and then around the vent. You can reach gently inside, moving your gloved fingers to the spine, and literally scoop out entrails in one move. If your chicken is large and your hands small you may need to reach in again to fetch heart and lungs at the front of the chicken's body. You're nearly done!

If you keep and use organs, remove the green bile sack from the liver (be certain not to cut into it) and tubes from the heart. Similarly, split the gizzard in half to remove the tough yellow lining. Wash and place neck, liver, heart, and gizzard into cold salted water while you finish the chicken.

If you've split and then cleaned out a chicken, you can freeze half birds for the barbeque or cut each half into individual pieces for the deep fryer. To butcher into pieces, use a boning knife at each joint for wings, thighs, and legs. Separating back from breast meat will require a closer cut with a carving knife.

Rinse the chicken inside and out, then immerse in slightly salted chilled water. When the temperature of the chicken has reached current air temperature or cooler, drip and pat dry, bag, and refrigerate for two days to age and tenderize. If you don't have room in your refrigerator you can place the bags directly into the freezer with similar results. Rotate your poultry two or three times a day for an even freeze.

Supplementary: Raising Turkeys

If you've ever eaten a homegrown turkey you'll never question a desire to feed one. So unlike the dry, almost sinewy, Christmas turkeys of the past, you'll swear it is an entirely different bird.

Personally—having eaten roast turkey dinner in more than thirty cooks' kitchens in forty years—I had never really enjoyed the meal. Until the day a farming friend served me the most delicious poultry I've ever tasted—a home-raised turkey.

A farm-raised turkey grows nearly as fast as a meat chicken and has similar feed-to-muscle conversion. They require no extra time (except in the first week) in chores and are easier to butcher, as feathers are fewer and the body cavity is larger. You can grow them to a family-appropriate size without worry of overgrowth and sparring among the male birds.

Growing white production breeds is the most common, as the finished bird has clean and bright skin with tender, short-fibered muscle. Large white hens are capable of reaching a fourteen- to sixteen-pound live weight in just four months. Toms will easily reach twenty-five to thirty pounds in five months. Dressed turkeys finish between 70 and 75 percent of their live weight.

Whether raising hens, toms, or a mix of both for three months, four square feet per bird is recommended. If growing on to five

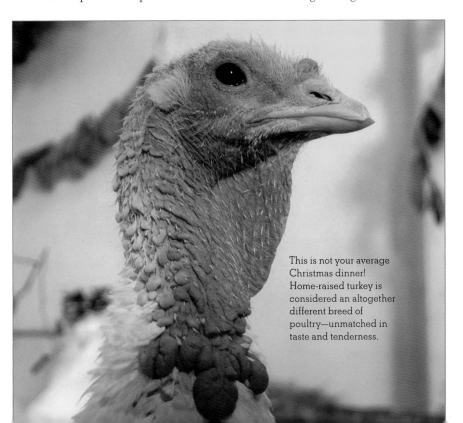

This is not your average Christmas dinner! Home-raised turkey is considered an altogether different breed of poultry—unmatched in taste and tenderness.

months, allow six or more. As always, my space recommenda-tions are slightly higher than industry standards. Increasing these numbers to 30 percent more floor space plus a fenced, protected, outdoor yard adds quality of life and creates tastier meat.

If you are already raising meat chickens you'll find it isn't much extra trouble to raise a few turkeys as well in your first year. A full wall partition separating the two will be required as turkeys are prone to picking up viruses from intermingling with chickens. This may sound like too much extra effort, but it is worthy work. By the time next spring rolls around you may just find yourself raising turkeys exclusively—especially if friends have been fortunate enough to share a meal with you! Prepare yourself. Once friends or family members have tasted this exquisite bird—the home-raised turkey—they will be asking you to raise some for them as well.

From Turkey Chick to Your Table

Consider the one- to fourteen-day-old turkey chick to be lacking in a survival instinct and you'll have no trouble raising them. They can drown in a quarter inch of drinking water. They can slip and fall and not figure out how to get back up. As lacking as they may appear in the first few weeks, by the time they've reached a month of age, their antics are less life-threatening and far more enter-taining.

During their stay with you they should always have easy access to fresh water and feed. They seldom make gluttons of themselves.

Day-old turkeys require perfection in their care. They are affected by chills and dampness, so their area must be 100 percent draft free and their water lukewarm. This is a chick that requires training on how to get a drink. Dip every beak, perhaps twice. To ensure they continue to find water, consider adding a few colorful marbles to their fount.

Turkey chicks aren't inquisitive by nature. They are, however, clumsy. Food needs to be easily available for the first three days and floor space should never be slippery. For the first three days cover their litter with an old sheet and sprinkle their feed on the surface. This ensures that they will not attempt to eat the litter and that they will be able to find their feed. Change the covering twice daily. By the fourth day all chicks know where the feeders are.

Turkeys will need a heat lamp providing temperatures of 95 to 105 degrees Fahrenheit for the first week. Turkey chicks will behave in the same manner as chickens—spending most of their time away from the light when temperature is adequate, huddling or stacking themselves on top of each other when they are cold. After the first week you can raise the lamp an inch or more to decrease floor temperature 5 degrees at a time. By five weeks of age they are capable of temperatures as low as 75 degrees, but if your nights are colder, keep the light on for another few weeks—if only through the night.

Turkey poults (sold at three weeks of age) are also available at most hatcheries. They'll cost twice as much or more, but are a bargain as they'll save you hours of heat lamp operation and have a lower mortality rate. Started poults arrive smart enough to find food and water.

Until they are eight weeks old, feed turkeys a commercial starter ration. I also purchase a vitamin powder to add to their water. Switch them to a grower ration until a few weeks before butchering, then switch them over to a finishing grain. You can slow down their growth if required by moving them to a finishing ration earlier and supplementing with oats, cracked corn, or turkey scratch grain.

More so than chickens, turkeys are susceptible to dampness, dirty litter, poor ventilation, chills, and overcrowding. If you're planning on raising turkeys, follow the guidelines in the earlier chapter on raising meat birds, paying special heed to preventing cannibalism. Slaughter and butchering practices also are the same as chickens.

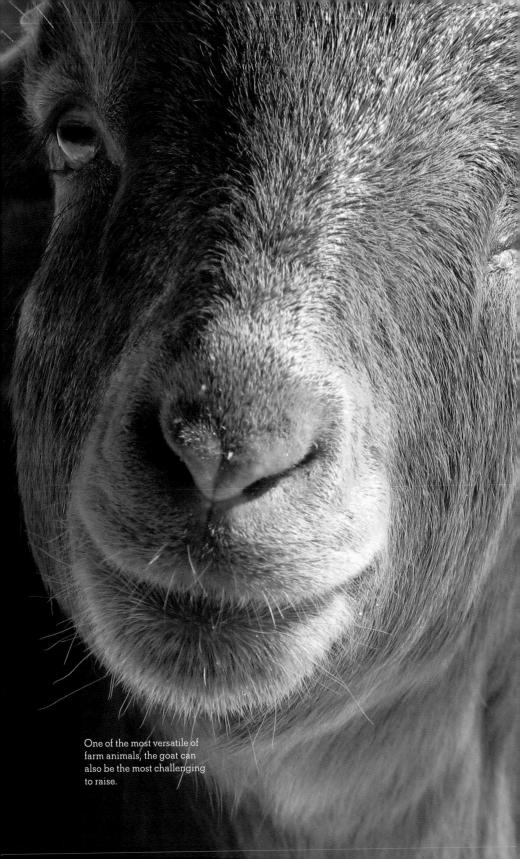

One of the most versatile of farm animals, the goat can also be the most challenging to raise.

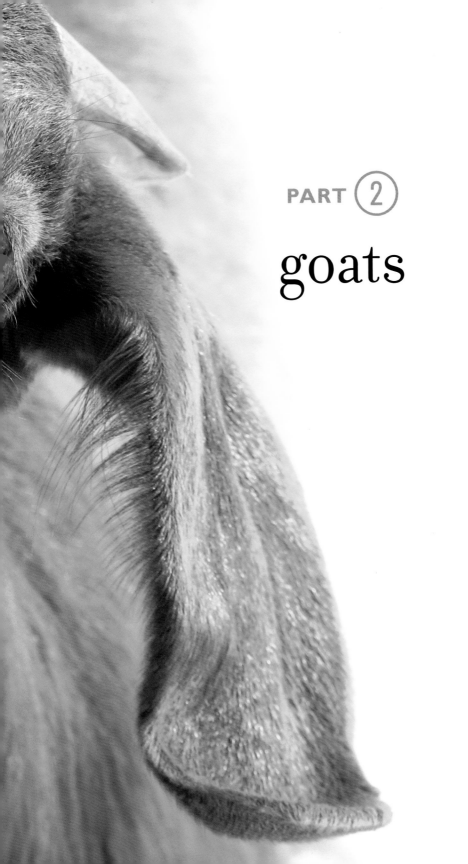

PART ②

goats

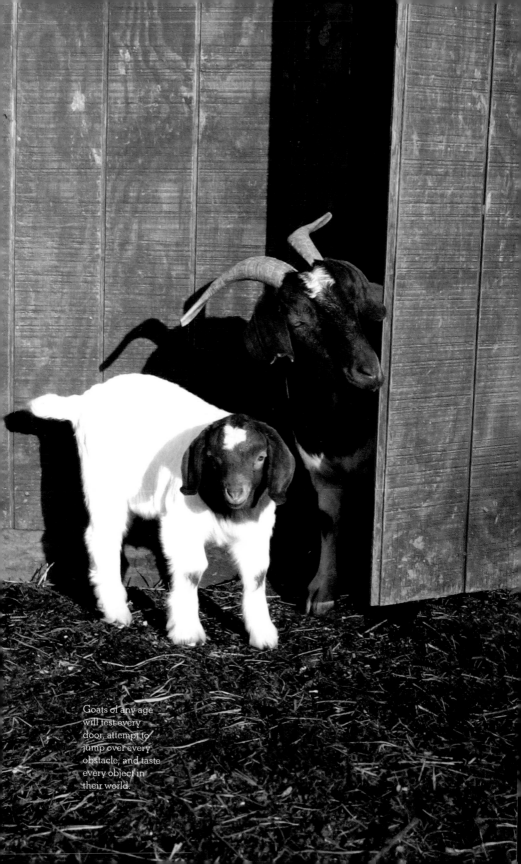

Goats of any age will test every door, attempt to jump over every obstacle, and taste every object in their world.

A goat, it has been said, is "like a three-year-old in a goat suit."

If you've ever thought you might like to try your hand at running a day care for preschoolers, you'll love looking after a few goats. They are both sweetness and shenanigans, loving and annoying, obedient and troublemakers—all within minutes of each other. They can double you over with laughter as easily as they make you cry out in absolute frustration.

With all the raw emotions that a goat or two can bring out in their keepers, they still count as the most versatile of all farm animals. With the right conditions one goat could supply your family with milk, low-fat meat, and an income throughout the year.

Milk from a backyard dairy goat can be used for household consumption and to make luxurious soaps. Although laws that allow the sale of milk are stringent, you could easily sell the soap as a high-end beauty product through multiple venues.

When compared to cow milk, goat milk is higher in phosphorous, riboflavin, niacin, calcium, and vitamins A and B1, and is lower in cholesterol. Right off the udder, goat milk is loaded with antibodies and has a much lower bacterial count than cow milk. Based on these and other benefits, goat milk is often recommended by doctors to safely treat physical conditions including eczema, vomiting (dyspepsia), and insomnia in infants, pregnant women, and children.

Goat milk is decidedly richer in flavor than cow milk if you are used to 1 or 2 percent milk from the grocer's shelves. As you'll see in the breed section (following) some goats produce milk that is up to 6 percent butterfat.

Although the milk may be high in fat, the meat from a goat is not. Found most often for sale within Spanish, Greek, and Jewish communities, chevon is growing in popularity across the United States and Canada. Chevon is the meat from a young, but mature, goat. Cabrito or chevrette is the term for meat from a milk-fed kid. The less tender meat from an older goat is called chivo or mutton (a term commonly used for older sheep meat).

Goats will give you much more than milk and meat though. You might be able to sell the hair from your goats or use them to control overgrowth on your land. A goat or two can make short work of returning a neglected homestead to its former beauty.

Measured by all these benefits, goats are a surprisingly inexpensive purchase and are also cheap to keep.

A final blessing of keeping goats is the fiber many of the breeds produce, known as cashmere. Cashmere is still the lightest weight, warmest, and most completely non-irritating fiber known to man. This down-like hair grows under the primary hairs of goats raised in cold climates where extra warmth is required. In most cases a cashmere-producing goat will only create a quarter to a third of a pound per year.

Dispelling Myths About Goats

Goats Are Smelly. Does smell like pasture, fresh air, and hay. It is the buck that carries the offensive odor that gives goats a bad name. Bucks have two major scent glands located slightly behind and between the horn area. The odor is strongest during breeding season.

Goats Are Mean. As a rule, goats are not mean. When raised with understanding and care they develop an eagerness to please their owners. Goats can be trained to come to their name, pull a cart or field tiller, and be led peacefully by a rope. If you've met a mean goat, you've either been in the presence of an uncaring owner or somehow the goat felt threatened and displayed aggression in an attempt to protect itself.

A Goat Will Eat Everything in Sight. Goats are inquisitive animals that explore their world orally. Few goats will swallow objects that don't taste good. Proper fencing is a top priority when raising goats to ensure they don't "explore" your prized roses or climb onto your pickup truck to see what's inside.

Choosing the Right Breed for Your Needs

Pure goat breeds are separated into three main groups for farm use—milk, meat, and fiber. A milk or fiber goat can be raised for meat. A meat or milk goat can produce salable fiber. Fiber and meat goats can be milked. Even though all goats are triple-blessed, not one breed is versatile or exceptional enough to be classified as such.

Around the world more than two hundred breeds of goat exist. Eighty of these are registered for agricultural use. The breed you choose will depend on your family's needs, your ultimate goal, and regional availability.

Approximately 60 percent of goats currently in North America are mixed breeds (termed "grades" or "scrubs"). These animals are unregistered but they still have use and purpose to a small farm. A grade goat might be a risky proposition to raise for milk, but they are perfectly acceptable animals for meat.

Meat, Milk, and Fiber Yields for Goats

Yields to be expected from registered classes are:

- Dairy—Average doe supplies nine hundred quarts per year.
- Meat—The average buck kid provides twenty-five to forty pounds of meat. Boer goats produce nearly twice as much.
- Fiber—Adult Angoras supply ten to fifteen pounds of mohair per year. Adult cashmere-producing goats might supply a third of a pound per year.
- All—Supply approximately one pound of garden-enhancing manure per day.

Dairy Goat Breeds

Of the six most common dairy goats, the Swiss breeds (Alpine, Oberhasli, Saanen, and Toggenburg) are the hardiest for colder climates. The remaining two (LaMancha and Nubian) are genetically equipped to handle extremely warm and dry climates but may be kept in the North with proper care and consideration.

Nubian—Easily recognized by long droopy ears and wide nostrils. Nubians are the most energetic class and produce milk high in butterfat.

LaMancha—These goats originated in the United States and have very small ears, if ears are at all noticeable. LaManchas are the calmest breed and also produce milk high in butterfat.

Saanen—The largest of the milk goats. Saanens are usually white, with a narrow face and nose. Saanens are one of the top two milk producers. Note: A colored Saanen is called a Sable. Although a Sable is the product of two Saanens with a present recessive gene,

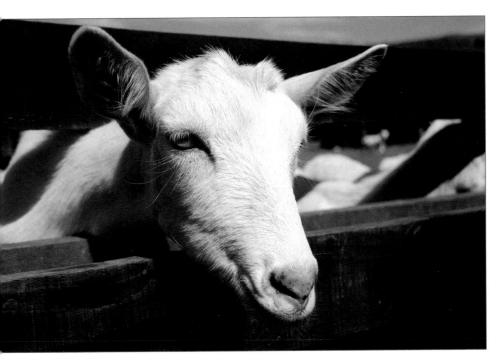

ABOVE: The Saanen is one of the top producing milk breeds.

Sables are slowly becoming recognized as a separate breed in North America.

Alpines—(French, Swiss, British, and Rock) Alpines come in a variety of colors, the most common of which is the French White Neck Alpine. These goats match the Saanens in milk production.

Toggenburg—Toggenburgs are the oldest registered breed. Usually brown (from creamy to dark brown) and showing white stripes or patches above each cheekbone, on the ears, inside the legs, and/or on the rump.

Oberhasli—You can easily see the genetic cousins of goats (deer) in the Oberhasli. These goats are small, like the Toggenburgs, and are easily distinguished by their thin faces and coats of russet brown, often with black markings.

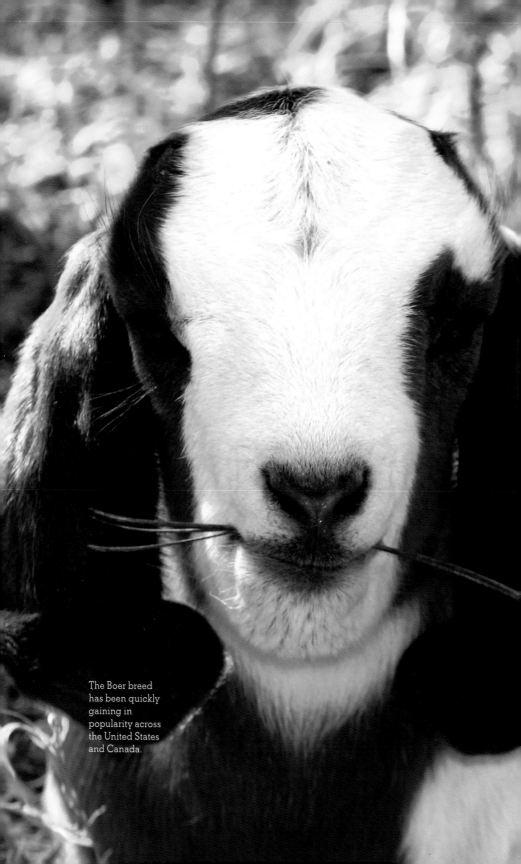

The Boer breed has been quickly gaining in popularity across the United States and Canada.

Meat Goat Breeds

Although any breed of goat (including the scrub) can be used for meat, this classification is specific to the few breeds that grow the quickest and add more lean muscle fiber than other classifications of goats.

The Spanish and Myotonic goats have been raised for centuries by North American farmers to provide a reliable meat source for their families. Both breeds grow to decent proportions and are well-muscled animals. Spanish bucks grow to an average of 175 pounds and their partners to 100 pounds. Myotonic bucks can weigh up to 140 pounds and the does approximately 75 pounds at maturity.

The Myotonic goat is also known as the Tennessee fainting goat. This goat was introduced into America by a Nova Scotian (Canadian) breeder. The animal's success as well as its shortcoming is the result of a genetic disorder causing it to react to fright with muscle spasms. The goat, when startled, will stiffen his legs, lose his balance in the process, and fall to the ground. The repeated stiffening gives the goat muscular thighs—enough so to be classified as a meat goat. Unfortunately this condition also renders the animal helpless in the pasture until the myotonia dissipates.

In the last century a new breed has entered North American soils. This breed, the Boer, hails from South Africa, where it was developed for size, speed of growth, meat quality, and uniformity of coat color. The Boer is statuesque in comparison to the native North American goats. A mature buck can tip the scales at more than 300 pounds, a doe at 220 pounds.

With a history and development similar to the Boer's, another new breed of meat goat is being introduced to the world from New Zealand. The Kiko goat is the product of a government-funded initiative that began in the 1970s to crossbreed wild with domestic goats to produce a faster-growing meat breed. Within just a few generations and minor variations during development, the Kiko was established as a breed. Kikos are now proven to have the highest occurrence of kidding twins, a fast and reliable growth rate, and a hardiness to disease and harsh weather.

Fiber Goats

Goats produce two distinct fibers—mohair and cashmere. While mohair is only produced by the Angora goat, cashmere can be found on more than sixty of the world's goat breeds. (In North America we most often find cashmere on northern-raised Spanish and Myotonic breeds.)

Finding a top-producing cashmere goat is difficult in North America, not to mention an expensive acquisition for the small herder. Goats in the top of their class for producing cashmere often net a few thousand dollars upon sale and yet may only produce a quarter to a third of a pound of fiber per year.

Angoras, on the other hand, are a pure and registered breed. These silky-haired goats generate eight to twelve pounds of mohair annually. A wether (castrated male) produces slightly more than a doe.

The Angora is certainly in a class of its own, but the care is similar to that of other goat breeds. If you are only planning on keeping a few and hope to sell the fiber twice a year, find a local breeder or Angora goat group to collaborate with. Not only will they share invaluable breeding, feeding, and coat care tips, they will also assist you in finding a buyer for your yield.

Miniature Breeds

Miniatures are currently popular on farms with limited space for both meat and milk production. The miniatures also make great pets and are easy enough for most children to handle. These goats are one-third to two-thirds the size of an average milk goat and therefore require much less space and food.

Nigerian Dwarf—At seventeen to twenty inches tall, this miniature dairy goat is capable of producing one quart of milk per day (ample for a small family) and requires a third of the space and feed that a full-size milk goat requires. Mature does average thirty to fifty pounds. Bucks and wethers average thirty-five to sixty pounds.

African Pygmy—These well-natured dual-purpose goats are often displayed at petting zoos. They stand eighteen to twenty-four inches tall, but their stocky build weighs them in at between thirty-five and seventy pounds. Their milk is higher in butterfat than any other goat (approximately 6 percent), and their muscular nature makes them a viable meat breed as well.

Although there are only two recognized miniatures, a few crossbreeds are gaining in popularity. The Pygora (a cross between an Angora and a Pygmy) produces a lesser-grade mohair but will also produce the fine down a Pygmy provides, and will finish a little larger for freezer meat.

Another dual-purpose crossbreed is the Kinder (a cross between a Pygmy and a Nubian). This breed has been gaining in popularity since first introduction in 1986. Kinders have been recorded to produce three to six kids annually, and some have been rated as top performing milkers (see the description of top performing milkers on page 77).

Designing Your Small Farm Strategy

As goats are herd animals, it is best to have more than one. They are not meant to be the only one of their kind on a farm, but they will bond and make friends with any other four-legged farm animal with which you house them. At any rate, if one is a charming addition to your farm, two will be twice the fun.

There are many options to consider when designing a small farm strategy to suit your needs. A few scenarios follow.

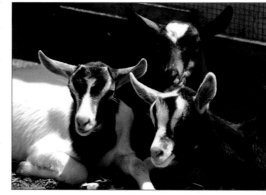

- Raise dairy goats with the added benefit of meat once per year: Purchase two bred or breeding dairy does. Breed them every year, four to six months apart from each other, to keep the milk flowing. Increase your herd by keeping the doelings or fill your freezer by growing the bucklings on supplemented pasture for four to six months. If you don't intend to increase your herd and your original does are of good stock, you can sell the young dairy does to other farms.
- Raise goats for meat and a little milk: Purchase two bred does of any breed (or have them bred) and continue to breed for the next few years. Keep or grow doelings and grow the bucklings for a few months.
- Raise goats for meat only: Purchase two wethers. Boer or Boer-cross wethers will yield the most meat in the shortest possible time.
- Raise goats for fiber with no interest in breeding or a milk supply: Purchase and keep wethers long-term. Wethers yield a higher fiber count, are cheaper to purchase, and grow larger than a doe.
- Raise Angora goats for income or for meat: Purchase two bred does, raise the offspring on supplemented pasture for meat, have some milk for personal use, and during shearing season make a little extra income.

Raising Kids for Meat

One of the most popular small farm strategies involves breeding milk does to keep them in production and raising the kids for just a few months to supply meat for the freezer. Others purchase weaned kids to raise for meat and are done with chores by winter solstice.

Whichever strategy you employ, your goal is to raise the largest possible kid, in the shortest period of time, at the lowest possible cost. The least expensive goat meat to raise is the six- to eight-week-old milk-fed kid weighing about thirty-five pounds. Since this kid will only net fifteen to twenty pounds of freezer meat, grow him on for a larger yield. By twelve weeks of age the average goat will weigh fifty pounds and will have only cost you a few dollars in grain. Put that same kid on pasture (with normal supplemental feeding), and by the time he's reached seven to eight months he should weigh in at eighty pounds.

Just by adding an extra five months of pasture grazing and a few pounds of grain, you've increased your freezer meat profit by 400 percent. The exception to this rule of increase is the Boer goat. Boers are larger at birth and grow faster and larger than any other goat in the same amount of time.

The Goat Barn, Yard, and Pasture

Whenever you need to set up an area for goats—inside or out—it is beneficial to remember the adage of a goat, "like a three-year-old in a goat suit."

If a barrier can be jumped over, an electrical wire reached, glass windows pushed upon, grain accessed, or nails stepped on, it will be. Any object within reach will be challenged, broken, eaten, chewed, ripped, pushed, or punctured by a goat. If you wouldn't leave your three-year-old nephew alone for twenty minutes in the shelter or hope to hold him with the fence you just built, it probably isn't adequate for a goat either.

Goats won't take up much room on your farm. Their housing requirements are nearly as casual as those required for chickens. In fact, a large shed will do just fine for a few goats. With just a little ingenuity and room in your budget you can have the ideal setup for keeping goats.

There are two primary methods for housing and containing goats. The first is to pasture them and provide a poor-weather and bedding shelter. The other method, "loafing and confinement," is to keep goats in a shed or small barn with a fenced yard for exercise.

The loafing-and-confinement system of raising goats is used mainly for dairy and fiber goats or by farmers who don't have ample pasture. Sufficient room is provided inside and out but keeps high-energy activity to a minimum. Less energy expended allows for productive use of feed.

An average goat only requires twenty square feet indoors, plus two hundred square feet outdoors. Meat goats require more: thirty square feet inside, three hundred outside. Miniatures require a third less than the others.

The Goat Barn

An existing shed conversion may be perfect for housing goats and could save you building a new structure. Knowing the number of goats you will house at the height of the season (your does plus offspring that you keep for five to six months) will determine if an existing building is adequate. A communal stall takes 35 to 50 percent of your floor space and leaves adequate room for a milking station, feed storage, and one or more smaller stalls. The small stall will be used for isolation of a sick goat, quarantining a new goat, kidding, or weaning.

Shed Conversion Example

Two dairy does given forty square feet (twenty square feet each) for a communal stall, plus a smaller stall for kidding (twenty square feet), a section for milking and grain storage (thirty-five square feet), plus twenty square feet extra for two kids annually.

At less than 120 square feet required, a little planning can convert a 10-foot by 12-foot shed into an adequate loafing barn. Tight, but adequate.

Design your floor layout to accommodate the feeding and watering of goats without entering their communal stall. The easiest way to do so is to build a half wall between their space and yours. Your side contains the manger, water bucket, and soda/salt feeder. Their side contains slatted or keyholed head access to all three.

A slatted or keyholed access manger may be the most economical investment of your time in a shed conversion. Goats

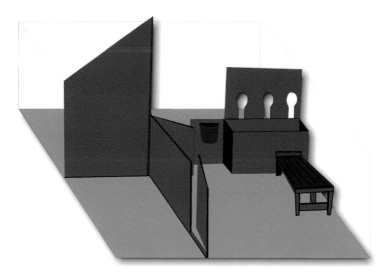

ABOVE: A converted ten-foot by twelve-foot shed showing a milking stand or bench, keyhole manger access, exterior water buckets, and good distribution of space: Sixty-square-foot communal stall, twenty-square-foot kidding stall, and thirty-five square feet of work and storage area. Add an access door to the back wall that opens to their yard and you're all set to bring a few goats home!

are not only notoriously picky about the hay they eat, they are also the most wasteful. If they can climb into a manger to eat they will do so, soiling their feed in the process.

At an open manger they are known for taking a mouthful of food, turning to see who might be behind them, and dropping half of their mouthful on the floor in the process. A slatted or keyholed access manger ensures that they can neither swing their heads around nor climb into the manger to eat.

The standard top width of a keyhole is eight to nine inches with a keyhole-shaped taper to the bottom at four to five inches wide. The full height of the keyhole is sixteen inches. Goats will crane their necks to put their heads in at the top and then lower their heads to a comfortable fit within the slot.

If the top of your wall is higher than most of your goats can reach through slats or keyholes, you could build a variable-height step on their side of the wall. Later, kids feeding at the manger will use the higher steps. Keyhole entries won't work for horned goats.

Temperature

Goats will huddle together and keep each other warm (enduring temperatures to freezing) as long as their goat house is free of drafts and leaks and the bedding is ample and dry. Take extra care for extremely cold days and nights, if kidding is imminent, or if you've had early-season births. Extra bedding, a supervised or safe heating unit, and/or a little extra hay for adult goats will help keep the cold out of your herd.

During the summer months you'll find goats equally resilient, but do not lock them in during the hottest summer nights without a breeze blowing through and plenty of cool water.

Floors and Bedding

The flooring in a goat barn need be nothing more than dirt covered with a thick layer of bedding material. Straw and waste hay are easy to use and inexpensive, but wood shavings are easier for cleaning and more beneficial as a future compost.

Keeping a goat's bedding clean is of the utmost importance. You won't have to spend hours cleaning out their pen every morning, though. All that is required is to lay some fresh bedding over the existing every few days.

When you're cleaning out the stall, be sure to compost the rich organic waste material for at least six months, then add it to your gardens. Compost longer if you've been using waste hay as bedding material.

Lighting

As the days grow short over the winter months, you'll find yourself doing chores in the dark more than once. If you keep dairy goats the addition of lighting performs double duty. Natural and artificial lighting for eighteen to twenty hours per day will maintain milk production through the fall and winter months plus increase the success rates of early spring breeding.

Grain or Goat Ration Storage

Store grain away from all moisture, out of the sun, off the ground, and certainly out of a goat's reach. Should a goat obtain access to the grain barrel it will eat until the grain is gone—gluttony that could result in death through bloat. A galvanized trash can with a snap-on lid placed well out of reach keeps goats and vermin out of the grain.

The Yard

The goat yard should be dry at all times to prevent bacterial infections in hooves. If you don't have a dry area available for goats, a poured concrete pad suffices during the rainy season. It will also keep their hooves neat and trim. Plan for at least part of the yard to be on the south side of the building.

Goats are happiest when they have something to climb on. An outcropping of rocks is ideal, but any sturdy structure will satisfy their instinctual nature to climb. Keep climbing objects well away from the fence or they'll use them as steps to freedom.

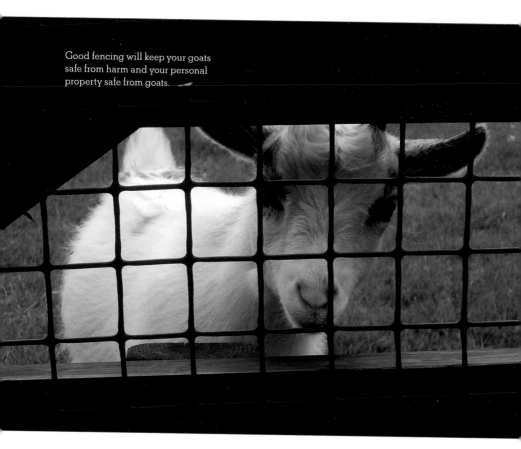

Good fencing will keep your goats safe from harm and your personal property safe from goats.

Fencing for Pasture or Yard

"A fence that can't hold water won't hold a goat" is an age-old axiom. Above all other considerations, the fence deserves the most attention. Goats will go over, under, or through a fence before you've taken three steps away from their yard if it hasn't been built correctly.

- Four-feet-high minimum. Five feet high for the highly active and nimble Nubians and miniature breeds.
- Page wire fencing with twelve-inch openings is acceptable if you will never need to contain kids; otherwise invest in a six-inch page wire. Chain link or stock panels with small openings are equally acceptable.
- Use eight-foot posts, eight to ten feet apart, buried at least thirty inches into the ground. Posts can be steel or wood.
- All corner post supports of a goat yard fence go on the outside. Goats will climb or shimmy up a fence support no matter how slim.
- If building an electric fence only, run the wire, from the bottom up, at five, ten, sixteen, twenty-three, and thirty-one inches, and a final strand at forty inches for all breeds. Electric fencing is not a viable option if power in your area is prone to blackouts, although you can also consider solar-powered electric fence chargers. They are common, effective, and not too expensive. Remove all weeds that touch the wire.

The Gate

Your goats will watch you enter and leave the yard. In doing so they will learn how to operate the lock. As soon as they've mastered the latch or handle they'll be wandering through your flower garden, investigating activity on the road, taking their lunch in the grain fields, or bleating at your front door.

A goat can flip a hook out of the eye it rests in and has the determination to mouth and hoof at a lever latch all day until it opens. Determined goats have even been known to slide a large bolt to the open position.

- Place all slide bolts, latches, or locks on the outside of the gate where the goat can't reach them.
- Install your gate to swing into the goat yard so that even if one of your escape artists managed to unlatch the gate, she might not know she did so.

The Pasture

The practice of pasturing goats is a personal decision that may be based on breed of goats, farm economics, available pasture, or even your need to have brush cleared on acreage.

As feed can be 70 percent of the cost of keeping any goat, even partially pasturing meat breeds is frugal and wise. Milking does set to managed pasture will create more milk, but it will be lower in butterfat content.

If you will be pasturing your dairy goats, take heed that consumed pungent plants could alter the flavor of milk. Ensure as well that the does aren't in forest or overgrowth. A milk goat's udder could easily be scratched or damaged while foraging in such conditions.

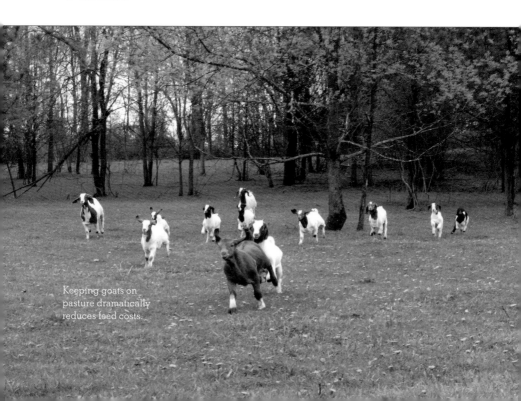

Keeping goats on pasture dramatically reduces feed costs.

Allow at least one acre for every ten goats and employ rotational pasturing by moving their pasture as soon as each area looks sparse. Rotating ensures that each pasture remains viable and decreases the potential for parasitic infestation.

Goats eat a wide range of native plants on acreage, but should still have access to free-choice hay so that they are not forced to eat less than desirable forage. Your goat may have an instinctual nature not to ingest harmful plants, but take precautions by walking your pasture and knowing the plants growing in it. Local authorities maintain lists of known poisonous plants in your region. Even nonpoisonous plants can be toxic if they've been sprayed with pesticides that are not within the realm of instinctual knowledge.

Goats on pasture, like any other animal, may be stalked and attacked by predators. Losing a prized goat or kid to coyotes, feral dogs, wolves, cougars, bears, and the like is heartbreaking. No two situations are alike in the most effective legal manner to cope with predators. Possible options for protecting goats might be a herd-protecting dog, donkey, or llama; stronger electric fencing; or hunting the predators. Always check local regulations before taking extreme action. Even though farmers have the right to protect their livestock, your problem predator might be a protected species.

Getting Your Goat

As you've already read, every goat needs a companion. This might as well be another goat, although a ewe, cow, or horse will suffice.

If a particular goat hasn't already caught your eye and captured your heart, it's time find the best stock that suits both the goat shed you've created and your budget.

One of the best places to find local breeders and receive third-party opinions is your feed supply store. The cashier or staff in these stores know the people who purchase goat ration and medications. They are generally happy to help a potential new customer and offer their opinion in the same breath. Just one name and phone number could open up an entire network of nearby breeders and goat husbandry associations for you.

While you are at the feed store, check the bulletin board—every feed store has one—for advertisements. If no such listing exists, become proactive and write up a quick "Goats Wanted" flyer and post it on the bulletin board before you leave.

Other viable options are the local classifieds, livestock auctions, and county fairs. Over the last few years, the Internet has grown enough to find nearby breeders or associations through any search engine. Type in your state plus the breed you seek. You should find hundreds of listings and your goat as the result of just one click.

Before you head out to a livestock auction with an empty trailer, please read the next section on assessing goats to avoid costly mistakes. You may luck out and find a beautiful animal at the auction at a decent price, but there is a substantial margin for error for new farmers. If you haven't owned goats before, either take someone with you who that knows goats and specifically the breed you seek, or use your time at the auction to network with the men and women selling or buying goats.

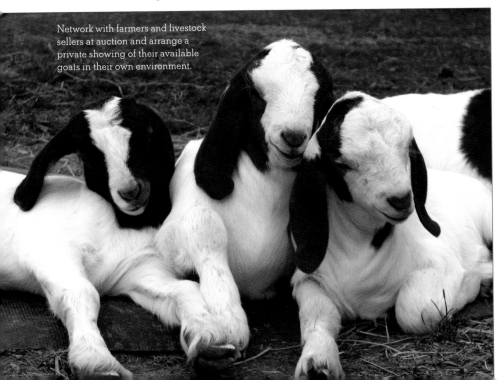

Network with farmers and livestock sellers at auction and arrange a private showing of their available goats in their own environment.

Most sellers are happy to arrange a private showing at their farm at a later date. Trade phone numbers and give them a call in a few days. Networking is, in fact, the better option. You'll make new friends who obviously share your interest and you might end up purchasing a special goat that a seller was apprehensive to sell to "just anyone." Viewing a goat in its comfort zone allows you to observe the breeder's housing arrangements and have ample time to chat and discuss registration, ancestry, and temperament, plus view any related barn records.

What to Look For

Price and paperwork aren't all there is to purchasing a goat. Health, age, production (even just in ancestry), and temperament are all key considerations.

Healthy, good-natured goats are easily handled and show neither shyness nor aggressive tendencies. Healthy goats will be as interested in you as you are in them. If she isn't looking at you with shining eyes and a sense of curiosity, you may want to move on to the next potential doe.

Know your breed. The body type should be a fair match to the breed you have chosen. Some goats have wide faces, some are without ears, others should fall within a certain height range by maturity. In all goats, look for a wide and strong back and chest, straight legs with trimmed hooves, and a clean, shiny coat. Avoid any goat with a sway back, a pot belly, bad feet, or a defective mouth.

The only way you'll develop an eye for healthy, productive goats is to closely observe as many of them you can. Whether you subscribe to a goat magazine, spend time at county livestock judging sessions, or discuss conformation with a local breeder, you will soon build up enough experience to be able to distinguish a strong, healthy animal from an unproductive underperformer.

Goat Registration Terminology

On the day you buy your goat you might hear some new terms from the private seller or auctioneer. Apart from doe (female), buck (male), wether (castrated male), and kid (not-yet-weaned offspring), here are some other descriptive terms.

Advanced Registry—Pertaining to milk does. This goat has been noted and registered as supplying a decent volume of milk over the course of a year. Dependent on their current age and health, Advanced Registry does have a proven record of milk production.

Star Milker—Pertaining to milk does. The star system is based on a one-day test of milk volume with extra stars awarded for ancestry performance. Points toward stars are calculated by a complicated formula used by goat dairies and registries.

Registered Purebred—Comes with a traceable pedigree (much like a purebred dog comes with registration papers and a family tree).

Grade—A grade goat may or may not be a purebred animal. It is without papers and registration. If your goat meets certain requirements and you desire it, you might be able to register it as a "recorded grade" with the issuing authority in your area.

Americans, Experimentals, NOAs—These are grade goats. Americans and Experimentals are certainly not purebred animals, but an NOA (native on appearance) might be.

Registered Goats Versus Grades

Although registration offers some reassurance that the animal you're buying is of notable heritage, it is not to be mistaken as a guarantee. A registered doe with an impressive ancestry may not be such an impressive milker. She might not even produce enough to keep the barn cat interested, or she may have trouble kidding, or both.

Registration papers matter most to those who plan to show, breed, or otherwise profit from the animals. If your strategy in raising goats is for personal use, the added expense and paperwork (now and in the future) are likely a waste of your resources.

Registration of a farm animal is similar to registration of a purebred dog—unnecessary for the average person's needs. You can look at a dog and tell whether it is purebred without seeing the paperwork. You can make general assumptions of production, personality, and growth rate based on the breed. For personal or farm use, a dog's registration is little more than paperwork to be shoved in a desk drawer.

The same theory holds true for goats. Some may disagree. They'll disagree vehemently when trying to sell you a goat out of your price range while waving registration papers in your face.

Somewhere on your adventure of keeping farm animals you'll discover your own comfort level and need for paperwork and registration. At the end of the day, no amount of registration beats trusting in the seller and your own ability to assess the age and health of an animal within reasonable doubt.

Keeping a Buck

You would do well never to keep a buck. Even though you will need to breed your milk does to keep their production up and your meat does to keep producing kids, there are better ways to accomplish the task than to keep a buck year round.

A buck requires separate housing, extra fencing, and twice as many chores. More often than not he is left in a shed of only adequate size and treated worse than a junkyard dog. Far too often I've visited or driven by farms and noticed unhappy bucks, isolated from all activity on the farm, in less than pleasant living quarters. Not only is this unfair to the animal, the buck's story almost always ends in grief. A buck all but ignored will eventually become too aggressive to handle at breeding time, and will become stressed due to his lonely living conditions. Stress decreases an animal's resistance to disease and does little for his breeding performance.

That same buck would be happiest on a larger farm with committed breeders who allow many does from many farms to be brought in for breeding.

Bringing Your New Goat Home

Any change in a goat's surroundings and routine will cause stress. Know your goat's current feed program (right down to the very hour) and bring a week's supply of her previous ration and hay home with her. For a few days don't alter her old routine. If you need to make changes, do so slowly over the course of a few weeks.

The seller should supply you with the following:

· Registration papers (if applicable)
· Veterinarian contact information
· List of past medications and vaccinations
· Feed (ration and hay supply) for the first transitional week
· Hooves trimmed and horn buds removed (if applicable)

Most sellers will worm the goat twenty-four hours before you pick her up. This ensures that she does not introduce worms onto your land. If the seller has not wormed her, do so while you keep her in quarantine.

Kid goats can be transported in a pet carrier or dog kennel in the back seat of your car. I have seen people transport full-size goats in the back seat of the family car, but I wouldn't do so unless the trip was twenty minutes or less and the route accommodated slow speeds.

The back of a pickup truck with a cap is perfect for transporting goats if you don't own a livestock trailer. Add three to four inches of straw, cover any metal loops or clasps, and you're set for the ride home. Take it easy on the turns and curves, and if your drive is longer than an hour, stop and check on the goat from time to time.

Quarantine any new goat for a week until the new surroundings become familiar and worming medication (if appropriate) has worked its way through her system. Slowly switch the feed over to your standard feed and spend plenty of one-on-one time with the new goat.

Feeding Goats

Goats are classified as ruminants and belong to the Bovidae family. They have a four-part stomach and will both graze pasture and browse woodland and brush.

In the wild, goats will eat leaves, branches, bushes, brush, and tree bark. They enjoy variety in their food and would rather reach up than chow down. Your goat may or may not have an instinctual ability to stay away from poisonous plants.

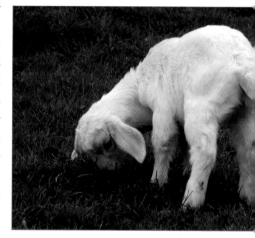

Contrary to popular belief, a goat will not eat everything in its path. Goats are prone to oral exploration and will mouth an object to experience it. Their interest in new adventures dictates that they must fully explore, rip at, tear apart, stand on, or conquer anything new to them. For their safety and that of your personal property, goats are not to be free-ranged around the homestead. Before you bring a goat home, take a look around and consider the potential trouble should they ever break free.

Feed Requirements

Goats require both hay (or pasture plus hay) and grain. If you are raising your goats for production you will want to be acutely aware of their nutritional needs and intake. You cannot assume a goat is fed nutritiously simply because it has filled up on brush, is on pasture, or has been given free-choice hay.

Goat ration is readily available at the feed store. The label will disclose added nutrients and vitamins as well as a protein count. A milking doe, for instance, requires 16 percent protein in her diet, while meat goats and wethers only require 12 percent.

Other nutrients may be required through supplemental feed. A prime example is selenium, a trace element required for the health of grazing animals but which has been depleted from the soil in some regions of the United States and Canada. Many feed manufacturers are aware of local depletion and have made up for this by adding selenium as a supplement to goat ration. Pay close attention to the labels and by all means collaborate with local herd owners or associations regarding supplemental nutrients.

Hay

Healthy goats won't eat more than they require. Keep free-choice hay available at all times even when your goats are on pasture. A belly full of fresh pasture and nothing else could result in fermentation, excess gas, and the potentially life-threatening condition of bloat.

The average goat eats 3 percent of her body weight in hay each day. Based on an average square bale weighing 35 to 40 pounds and an average goat weighing 120 pounds, you'll need approximately thirty-five to forty square bales of hay per year, per goat.

Kids and pregnant or lactating does will benefit from a higher-legume hay if you can find it. Legume hays are alfalfa, clover, soybean, vetch, and lespedza. Hay that is adequate for cows will not provide enough nutrients for goats. Cow hay is just barely suitable as bedding for a goat. You need hay fit for a horse or better. A 50-50 ratio of legume to grass is perfect.

The amount of hay you put out each morning or evening will vary through the seasons. It is completely normal for goats to eat the best part of the hay and leave half of the bale in the manger. Don't let old hay sit in the bottom of the manger. Rotate it for a day perhaps, then delegate waste hay to bedding.

When you're keeping goats, the biblical idiom "make hay while the sun shines" is changed to "store hay while the sun shines" for farmers on a budget. With two goats to care for you'll be using eighty bales of hay throughout the year. Storing it on your own property as soon as it comes off the farmer's field is both economical and wise. You don't want to be scrambling for hay in February, paying a higher price per bale, and worrying about moving it around during freezing weather.

Ration

Every goat requires grain for good health, and goats in production even more so. Nutritionally designed goat ration (also called goat chow) exists to match a goat's age, breed, purpose, and current condition. Every goat type, in fact every goat in your herd, will require a different amount of ration per day. Use the chart below as a starting point to determine your goat's needs, then adjust quantities based on physical condition, seasonal changes, and the quality of hay you're currently feeding. With minor adjustments throughout the year you will find the perfect quantity for every goat in your barn.

General Ration Guidelines for Goats		
Type	**Condition**	**Daily Amount (in pounds)**
Kid	Nursing	If interested, a bite or two
	Weaned on pasture	1/4–1/2
	Weaned no pasture	1
Wethers/Open Dry Does		1/2 (maintenance)
Non-Dairy Does	Bred and Dry	1/2–1 (maintenance)
	6 weeks before kidding	1 (concentrate)
	Nursing	1–1 1/4 (concentrate)
	12 weeks after kidding	1/2–1 (maintenance)
Dairy Does	Bred and Dry	1 (concentrate)
	2 weeks before kidding	Up to 3 (concentrate)
	Lactating	1 plus 1/2 per pound of milk produced (concentrate)

Some quick adjustment guidelines per individual goats are:

- Decrease ration to goats on pasture, overweight goats, wethers, and dry (non-lactating) does.

- Increase ration to recently weaned kids, underweight goats, goats on pasture in bad weather, and pregnant or lactating does.

Water

Your goat needs fresh, clean water accessible at all times. No exceptions. The quantity goats consume will change with the seasons, their condition, and their present food supply. On average, one goat will consume one to four gallons per day.

As with hay, the best way to supply goats with water is head access only. Place water buckets outside of their pens where they cannot spill or soil them, but can easily get a drink. Empty and replenish water buckets daily, then sanitize weekly to prevent bacteria-related illnesses.

Extra Supplementation

Goats need a low level of acidity in their four-part stomach to maintain proper digestion. Grain and rich pasture may increase acidity and upset the balance. Increased levels of fermentation could prove fatal to a goat. Given the correct supplementary aids, a goat self-manages its acidic range without further intervention. Access to soda and salt is all that is required.

The average goat will consume two tablespoons of soda per day. Feed-grade baking soda is available at your feed store, but the grocery store version will get you through until your next visit to the feed store without harming a goat (it just costs more).

Salt is available in block form as well as loose. Request a trace mineral salt mix formulated specifically for goats. If not available, horse or cow salt mixes can be appropriate if they contain copper, iodine, and selenium (in regions that are depleted). Staff at the feed store or your veterinarian will know if your region is high or low in selenium and other trace minerals and if extra supplementation is required. Unlike excess protein, which harmlessly flows right through a goat, excess minerals can upset a goat's healthy balance.

Maintaining Good Health in Your Herd

A goat can be kept healthy for most of her life by following standard barn practices of cleanliness, maintenance, and prevention. There will be times, though, when the cause of illness is so minimally within your control that you couldn't have prevented it and your goat gets sick. Opportunities for the introductions of illness, parasites, toxic reactions, and bacterial infections are everywhere on a farm—there is no way around it. Learn to recognize the warning signs and take appropriate action when necessary. In my opinion, being over-protective of animals in your care is not a character flaw.

First Aid Kit

It took me a full year to wise up to the fact that keeping supplies and notes in a barn was a good idea. After multiple trips to the house and back gathering supplies to treat my animals, I eventually assembled a first aid kit for the barn. Once you've raised goats for a few years you'll have your own favorites to keep on hand, but to get you started, here are the contents of my own kit:

- Rectal thermometer and isopropyl alcohol (to sterilize it)
- Three clean towels wrapped individually in plastic bags (to keep them clean)
- Antibiotic ointment
- Udder balm (for chapped udders)
- Deworming medication (watch the expiration date!)
- Hydrogen peroxide
- Tetanus antitoxin
- Mineral oil (for bloat)
- Propylene glycol (for doe ketosis)
- Electrolyte powder (for dehydrated kids)

Although you may not be one for keeping notes (and to be honest neither am I), forcing yourself to keep a barn journal may one day save your goat's life. A reference of a goat's change in eating habits, energy levels, or appearance is the best tool you can hand a veterinarian called in for diagnosis and treatment.

Barn records serve a secondary purpose. If you are ever called away or can't get back home to do chores, any friend or neighbor armed with these records could walk into your barn and take over with minimal risk of adverse effects.

For each animal you might record daily ration amount, daily milk given, changes in eating habits, quarterly weight and temperature, last breeding date, hoof trimming dates, and vaccination records. Although warning signs of illness vary, you'll know when your goat is not feeling up to par at a glance. Take note of the subtle changes and you may catch an illness, infection, or disease before it becomes life-threatening.

Any breeding herd should be vaccinated against enterotoxemia, chlamydiosis, and tetanus annually. If you vaccinate a doe four to six weeks before kidding, some immunity will be passed on to her kids. Based on your veterinarian's recommendation, you may also vaccinate four to six weeks before breeding. Kids should be vaccinated against enterotoxemia and tetanus at two months of age, followed by a booster a month later.

It is also good practice to treat your goats for worms in the fall and spring. This may also require your veterinarian's assistance. A fecal sample is submitted for assessment before treatment is prescribed or recommended.

Changes in Weight

Measuring and recording a goat's weight monthly is good barn practice. Weight is a benchmark used to measure health, preparation for breeding, kid development, and if ration amounts require adjustments. A sudden drop in weight is the earliest signal that health is waning.

Weigh your goat again before medicating for illness or treating for worms. Too much medication could cause an overdose; too little medication and the treatment won't be effective. To further complicate the matter, consistently underdosing literally trains organisms (bacteria and worms), to become resistant to the drug. Later on, even a corrected dosage will not be effective.

You can arrive at a quick approximation of weight using a measuring tape and the following chart. The measurement is taken from the goat's heart girth, the area directly behind the front legs. If you are weighing kids with a heart girth of less than eighteen inches, use a house scale to weigh yourself first, and then again with the kid in your arms. Subtract your weight from the combined weight and you'll have the kid's weight.

Signs of Illness

Your goat's mannerisms and appearance are the next telling signs of illness, infection, or disease. Some temperamental and physical warning signs might be:

· Lethargy
· Teeth grinding
· Coughing
· Shallow breathing
· Disinterest in ration
· Changes in manure color or consistency
· Change in milk color, quantity, or consistency
· Rough coat
· Dull eyes and/or change in color of the eye socket, gums, or facial skin (usually pink—watch for pigment changes to pale or blue)

Weight Chart for Large Breed Dairy Goats	
INCHES	POUNDS
18.25	23
19.25	27
20.25	31
21.25	35
22.25	39
23.25	43
24.25	51

Weight Chart for Large Breed Dairy Goats	
INCHES	POUNDS
25.25	57
26.25	63
27.25	69
28.25	75
29.25	81
30.25	87
31.25	93
32.25	101
33.25	110
34.25	120
35.25	130

Common Diseases and Illnesses

Some of the most common goat viruses and illnesses are listed on the following pages. For each listing I've tried to provide a preventive measure to help you maintain good health in your goats. In a few of the listings you'll find that there are no known cures or treatments. Please check with your veterinarian for recommendations on any animal's care. Cures and treatments are discovered every year, as are new diseases. If you have any concern over the health of a goat, take a temperature reading, isolate the animal in a quiet stall, and call the veterinarian.

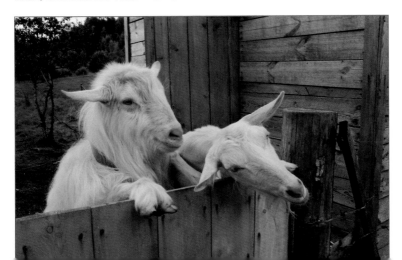

Common Illnesses

Abscess

Firm to hard fibrous lumps under the skin of an animal caused by a bacterial infection of the lymph nodes. Most bacterial infections resulting in an abscess can be traced back to a flesh wound.

Prevention: Provide the safest yard and house for your goats. Metal protrusions from the ground, fences, and barn walls can cut through a goat's hide.

Treatment: Isolate the goat from the herd and call the veterinarian to discuss severity. An expensive surgical operation might be required to remove the abscess.

Bloat

Bloat is a life-threatening, painful buildup of excess gas. If you see a growing swelling on the goat's left side and the goat is very restless, don't hesitate to place a call to the veterinarian's emergency number.

Prevention: A change in diet or too much ration is usually the culprit. Keep grain and ration well out of a goat's reach and introduce new foods slowly.

Treatment: While waiting for the veterinarian to arrive, try to keep the goat on its feet with the help of family, a wall of hay, or any other means. Rub the goat's stomach area to help move and alleviate gas buildup. Drench the goat orally with two cups of mineral oil and follow up with a half cup of baking soda dissolved in room temperature water. Do not attempt this if you've never given a goat oral medication before.

CAE/CAEV

This deadly virus—caprine arthritis encephalitis—is still without a cure. The virus is passed from one goat to another and is easily recognizable by swollen and stiff knee joints in mature goats and weak rear legs in kids.

Prevention: Have your goats tested for the virus annually. Only purchase goats that are certified clear. Quarantine any new additions for at least a month and have your vet test the animal before releasing into herd population.

Treatment: None.

Chlamydiosis (Chlamydial Abortion)

This deadly disease is contagious to humans. If you are assisting with a live birth, wear long plastic gloves and scrub thoroughly after kidding. Warning signs are a premature abortion during the final eight weeks of pregnancy. If the doe carries the kids to full term, they are either stillborn or very weak.

Prevention: Part of your vaccination schedule.

Treatment: None. Discuss each doe's future with your veterinarian and immediately remove affected does from the herd to prevent spreading the disease.

Coccidiosis

A potentially life-threatening parasitic infestation. You'll notice a lack of appetite and energy. Your goat may lose weight quickly or develop bloody droppings. Cause of coccidiosis is a protozoal parasite.

Prevention: Keep the goat house, feeders, and watering stations clean.

Treatment: Coccidiostat available at most feed stores or through your veterinarian.

Diarrhea/Scours

The trouble with scours and kids is that they will very quickly become dehydrated and too weak to feed. Scours are often brought on by a change in diet, but could be the signs of other problems.

Prevention: Keep the goat house, feeders, and watering stations clean. Pregnant does may be vaccinated to assist in the prevention of scour-causing illnesses.

Treatment: Isolate any kid with scours immediately. Disinfect every bit of your barn or goat shed. Call the veterinarian for advice and bottle-feed electrolyte fluids to any affected kid (available at the feed store) instead of milk ration for two days.

Enterotoxemia

Classified as a life-threatening bacterial infection. This condition is also called overeating disease. Goats are seen to twitch, show signs of bloat, grind their teeth (a sign of pain in goats), and have an increase of temperature.

Prevention: Part of your vaccination schedule. Avoid changes in diet.

Treatment: None.

Hoof Rot

If there were one good reason a goat's yard and bedding should always be dry, hoof rot would be it. This bacterial infection can result in death, but you'll notice it and have time to treat it well before that happens. Symptoms are smelly feet, lameness, loss of weight, and potentially tetanus.

Prevention: Trim hooves regularly. Keep bedding clean and yard dry.

Treatment: Trim away hoof to a consistent length and to healthy tissue. Soak the foot for two minutes in water with dissolved copper sulfate (at a ratio of one gallon water to one half pound copper sulfate, respectively). If the condition is severe, consult with your veterinarian for antibiotic treatment.

Internal Parasites and Worms

Repeated pasturing in one area without rotation is the main cause of repeated worm infestation. The goat consumes worm eggs in the grass, and they hatch and mate in the stomach and then lay eggs in the intestine. The eggs are released with every bowel movement, the grass grows, and the eggs are consumed again.

Although completely natural and an inescapable part of life, parasitic infestations can drag a goat's health down with poor appetite, coughing, reduction in or strange-tasting milk, and weight loss.

Prevention: Rotate pasture. Keep all feed and water dishes meticulously clean. Follow your veterinarian's suggested worming schedule based on available pasture and regional climate.

Treatment: Have your veterinarian test a fecal sample and provide medication.

Ketosis (Pregnancy Toxemia)

Ketosis is a metabolic disorder that could be life-threatening. Usually brought on by feed quality not matching a doe's condition (age, breed, weight, health) and her body starts giving of itself to facilitate fetal growth. Most often seen in does a few weeks prior to, or just after, kidding. The doe goes off her feed, may appear lame, and may have sweet-smelling breath or urine.

Prevention: Follow a responsible feeding schedule with bred does. Ensure that the feed supplied is of the highest quality and is offered free-choice. As fetal growth draws energy and nutrients from the doe, and less space is available within the doe's stomach, she cannot consume large amounts of feed at a given time. Does that were overweight before breeding and then fed a nutrient-lacking diet are more susceptible to ketosis, but it is also common in first-time mothers and does carrying multiples.

Treatment: If you catch ketosis in time (by noticing that the doe's not eating), add a feed-grade dry molasses to her ration or concentrate to entice her to eat. Separate her from the herd to monitor her fluid intake. You need to ensure she gets some type of energy (in the form of sugars such as molasses or propylene glycol) and sufficient water to flush the ketones out of her kidneys. Ketones are the byproduct of the doe's system metabolizing fat into glucose. If she worsens, call the veterinarian.

Lice

Consistent scratching and biting, loss of weight and hair, and decreased milk production could be warning signs of a lice infestation—especially if your goats are currently living in a damp environment.

Prevention: Keep living quarters dry and avoid contact with infested animals.

Treatment: Any powder, dip, spray, or pour-on insecticide approved for livestock or dairy animals will work and should all be available at your local feed store.

Mastitis

A painful bacterial udder infection for does. Your doe may stop eating. Her udder may be hard, swollen, or abnormally hot or cold. Her milk might smell bad or show signs of blood.

Prevention: Keep living quarters clean, dry, and safe. Apply a teat dip after every milking session. Once a month, check your does with a mastitis test available from your local feed store (dairy cattle tests work fine for goats).

Treatment: Based on your veterinarian's recommendation, antibiotics might be in order. Milk the doe three times a day to relieve pressure and apply hot packs to the udder four times a day. Isolate from herd. Dispose of her milk if antibiotics are used, and consult with the veterinarian for a clear date.

Orf

Also known as sore mouth, scabby mouth, contagious pustular dermatitis, and ecthyma. This viral condition causes thick scabby sores on the lips and mouths of kids and may last up to four weeks. Kids may have trouble nursing and as a result could suffer malnutrition. Nursing kids with orf can pass the infection onto the teats of a doe, which can quickly escalate into mastitis.

Your veterinarian may suggest quarantine of nursing kids with does and a sterilizing teat and udder wash four times per day for at least four weeks after the first signs of orf.

There is a human health risk associated with this virus. Wear rubber gloves and sterilize all equipment thoroughly.

Prevention: There is nothing you can do to prevent this virus.

Treatment: An after-infection, veterinarian-supervised vaccine is now available to prevent further incidence.

Pinkeye

Caused by bacteria or virus. Goats will squint and have watery eyes.

Prevention: Contagious. Avoid contact with infected goats.

Treatment: The entire herd should be treated with antibiotic drops.

Pneumonia

Various bacteria and viruses attack an already stressed or ill goat. May also be brought on by unrelated allergic reactions. Warning signs are coughing, loss of appetite, fever, and runny nose and eyes. Drafts and wet living conditions exacerbate the potential for pneumonia.

Prevention: Keep your goats as stress-free as possible. Ensure their housing is free of cold drafts.

Treatment: Call your veterinarian for antibiotic treatment.

Ringworm

Ringworm is brought on by fungi in the soil that attacks the skin of an animal. It shows up as circular skin discoloration resulting in hairless patches on the head, nose, neck, or udder.

Prevention: Highly contagious to both animals and humans. Avoid contact with infected animals.

Treatment: Wear rubber gloves and follow a strict sterilization practice. Scrub the patches with warm, soapy water and coat with iodine or fungicide available from your local feed store.

Scrapie

Scrapie is a neurological disease (similar in nature to mad cow disease) that has been under steady investigation since 1952 to determine cause and discover a cure.

Only seven cases have been reported in goats, and in all cases the disease has been acquired from contact with sheep. Further information on scrapie can be found in the sheep health section of this book, on the Internet at www.keepingfarmanimals .com, or (if in the United States) by calling the USDA Animal and Plant Health Inspection Service at (866) 873-2824.

Tetanus

Harmful bacteria enter through a flesh wound and create stiff and spasmodic muscles. Early warning signs are wide eyes and flared nostrils.

Prevention: Part of the kids' vaccination schedule at four weeks and then eight weeks of age.

Treatment: Detected early, tetanus can be halted with veterinary care and medication. Advanced cases are without cure and result in death.

Ticks

If your goats pasture and browse in wooded areas, ticks may be a problem—for both you and your goats. You may find them rubbing or scratching the tick's point of entry as well as losing hair and weight. Check forest-pastured goats daily during tick season in your region and remove any you find immediately.

Wounds

Goats are prone to cuts and scrapes due to their curious and adventurous nature. Although the cuts themselves aren't much of a problem, the introduction of diseases and infections through flesh wounds can be life-threatening. Knowing how to sanitize and treat those wounds immediately and routinely is a necessity.

Treatment: Clean the wound with hydrogen peroxide. Stop any bleeding by applying pressure with a clean towel. Clip hair around the wound and flush the area with warm, soapy water. Rinse with clear water to remove any soap residue, apply hydrogen peroxide once again, and cover the area with an antibiotic ointment. Every day check, clean, and redress the cut until it is fully healed. If the wound becomes infected, call your veterinarian immediately.

GOAT VITAL SIGNS AND GROWING CYCLE

- Rectal temperature: 101.5 to 105 degrees Fahrenheit
- Pulse rate: seventy to eighty beats per minute
- Breathing rate: twelve to twenty breaths per minute
- Puberty: At five months to a year of age, dependent on breed
- Average birth weight: eight pounds
- Average gestation period: 150 days
- Heat cycle: every eighteen to twenty-four days
- Heat period: approximately one day

Grooming

A hoof trim is one maintenance task that doesn't take much time but is absolutely necessary to your goat's health. Without proper hoof care your goat can become sick, lame, or permanently crippled. Frequent attention to hoof care, no matter how minor, is decidedly easier than infrequent major trimming. From the age of two months I make all goats stand and allow inspection, or a trim, of their hooves every month.

If you pasture your goats like I do (on somewhat rocky pasture) the hoof will wear down naturally, which minimizes the monthly task. Goats restricted to a small yard seldom have that opportunity, but the addition of a small concrete slab or a stack of large rocks to climb on will help them maintain their hooves and lighten your chore load.

To Trim a Hoof

Confine each goat in a manner that prevents escape. A dairy stand with stanchions, leash and collar tied to a barn wall or fence, or a helpful friend are all great ways to keep a goat confined for a few minutes. If your goat is being particularly difficult, lean your shoulder into her side with her other side against a wall while you work on each hoof. Angoras and kids can be "sat" on their rumps, leaning against your legs while you work.

Stay calm while you work and you will find that your goat remains calm as well.

- Wear gloves.
- Bring shears, a rasp, and hydrogen peroxide to the barn with you.
- Soft hooves are easier to trim than dry hooves. Allow your goats an hour in the yard, as hooves are softened by morning dew.

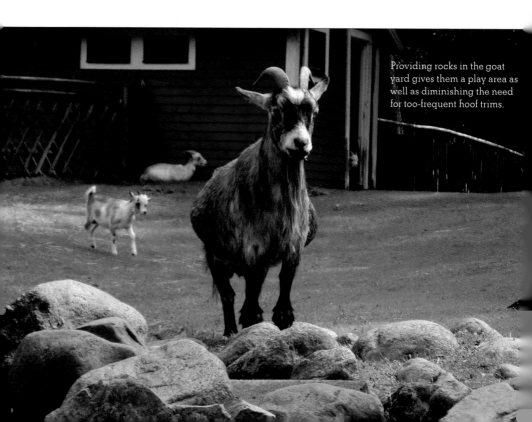

Providing rocks in the goat yard gives them a play area as well as diminishing the need for too-frequent hoof trims.

- Constrain the goat in a manner that allows you easily and comfortably to bend the goat's leg for observation of, and work on, the entire bottom of the hoof.

Step 1: Gently scrape out any impacted dirt in the curve of the hoof with a hoof pick or the point of closed shears. Work gently inside the wall. Impacted dirt at the toe of the hoof does not need to be forced out. Get the debris that falls out easily as you trim. It will all have fallen away by the time the hoof is trimmed.

Step 2: Snip away the overgrowth at the toe of the hoof (it will be the longest), then move on to the sides and remove any folds or excess found there. Your objective is a level foot—a hoof wall that just barely extends and protects the frog.

Step 3: Use a hoof rasp to create a smooth finish on the hoof wall.

Should a goat arrive on your farm with a severely overgrown hoof, only take a little off at a time every five to seven days. It may take a month, but eventually you will have a neat and trim hoof.

If you happen to snip too far and your goat bleeds, clean the wound with hydrogen peroxide and check daily for signs of infection.

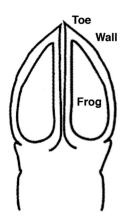

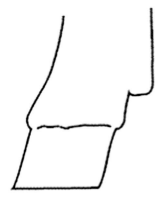

ABOVE LEFT: The anatomy of a hoof.

ABOVE RIGHT: A nicely trimmed foot. The base of the hoof is parallel to the coronary band (the area where the hair ends and the cuticle begins).

Gifts of Keeping Goats

Milk from a doe that has proper care tastes so similar to cow milk that most people would be hard-pressed to tell the difference. Even though only a fraction of North Americans know that goat milk is palatable, more people worldwide drink goat milk than any other milk.

In the milk industry, goat milk is never measured in gallons or quarts but by weight. Small herd farmers just keeping a few goats for personal use, however, continue to measure their daily supply in standard liquid measurements. A good milk doe can supply your home with nine hundred quarts of milk over the course of a year. Some dairy breeds are known to give milk that is rich in milk fats, making it perfect for creating a variety of cheeses in your own kitchen.

Milk Production Management Issues

A goat's milk production is dependent on the kidding cycle. Peak production is two months after kidding, but a good dairy goat continues to produce milk long after her kids are weaned.

When a doe first gives birth, her body begins producing milk. The term for this is "freshening." For the next eight weeks her supply increases, levels off for four months, and then begins decreasing until she is bred again.

Standard small-herd practice is to breed the milkers once per year, dry them out for two months previous to kidding, and breed them again. If you follow that strategy, most does will supply you with milk for 240 to 300 days of the year. If your doe dries out early—only supplying milk for eight months or so—she's still a good milker for any family.

Your doe will be at the height of her production in her fourth and fifth years. Negative factors affecting milk production are stress, insufficient natural or artificial lighting, weather, injury, feed quality, illness, or major disruptions in their routines. Milk does thrive on routine and goats require milking twice per day. You get to set the time, but for best results remain consistent with their schedule and keep milking sessions about twelve hours apart.

Equipment and Supplies for Milking Goats

Although you could get by in a pinch with a high-quality stainless steel bowl from your kitchen, a cheap milk strainer, and some quart canning jars, you will be milking twice a day for at least 250 days a year, so you might as well have the proper equipment.

Equipment for Milking

- Milk stand (with or without stanchions)
- Clippers and a brush to trim and brush hair away from back, sides, and udders to prevent hairs shaking down into the milk
- Udder wash to remove any debris and to sanitize hands
- Small bowl or mug used as a strip cup (squirt in the first milk from each teat for a visual quality check.)
- Stainless steel milk pail
- A made-for-goats teat dip to prevent bacterial infections
- Bag balm (to prevent chafing or chapping of the udder and teats)
- Notebook to record milk amount from every session
- Dairy strainer with disposable milk filters
- Milk scale for weighing milk per session (I don't personally use these.)
- Home pasteurizer (pasteurize milk yourself with a double boiler and a candy thermometer. Heat milk to 165 degrees Fahrenheit and maintain for 30 seconds.)
- Glass milk jars
- Chlorine bleach
- Stiff-bristle (plastic) brush
- Dairy acid cleaner

A relatively skilled carpenter can create a simple milking stand including stanchions in just a few hours and with less than one hundred dollars' worth of lumber. Goat stanchions can also be purchased online—new or used.

Sanitizing Equipment

Sanitize all equipment before and after milking, including udder, teats, and hands, to ensure a healthy, happy doe and high-quality milk.

To sanitize equipment between uses, first rinse in warm water to remove fat residue. Next scrub with a bristle brush using hot water, dish detergent, and an ounce of chlorine bleach. Rinse in clear water and then in a dairy acid cleaner. Never use dishcloths to wash or towels to dry. These items, even fresh out of the laundry, are loaded with bacteria. Allow your equipment to drip dry.

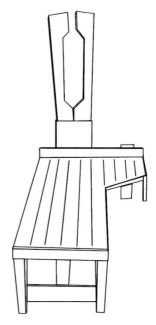

ABOVE: A homemade milking stand offers stanchions (to hold the goat's head in place), a sturdy stand for the goat, and even a small sitting area for the milker.

How to Milk a Goat

When it comes right down to brass tacks, farmers have been milking goats for centuries without all the fancy equipment. I'm half embarrassed to tell you my own story, but I want to make a point about getting by with what you have. Picture this: A doe and her needing-to-be-weaned kid landed in my barn and I, knowing nothing other than the rules of sanitation and pasteurization, proceeded to milk her twice daily.

She was young and small, and in retrospect I guess she had been bred too young. This worked in our favor, though, as she had never given milk and I had never taken it. She would not stand idly on the barn floor and let me milk her. I had never heard of a stanchion, but I was determined that she stand without fussing or kicking over the bucket. The only way I could hold her in place by myself was to lock her head between my legs, bend forward across her back, and milk her. I did this twice a day, every day, for a month before I started asking around for advice.

Although that method is neither conventional, efficient, nor 100 percent effective, we still drank healthy, delicious milk every day. Today I have a milking stand.

The Milking Process

There is a rhythm to milking a doe. You can learn it just by watching the kids. Bump. Lock. Draw.

Once you have positioned your doe, prepare her for a milking session by brushing her coat to prevent hair from dropping into the milk pail and wash her udder and teats with a teat dip. With your milk pail in place, lock your forefinger and thumb around a teat at the base of the udder and draw down. Never squeeze her udder, only her teat.

There will be milk waiting in the teat, which you will guide out with a squeeze, *drawing* downward, not *pulling* downward. If the difference doesn't make immediate sense to you, think of how you might squeeze all of the toothpaste out of the tube with only one hand. Better yet, imagine guiding your doe's milk along a straw, softly pushing it down, one finger tightening at a time.

After a full draw down and into the bucket, release the pressure on your top two fingers to allow more milk to enter the teat, and draw again. Release. Each time that you release your grasp the teat fills up with milk again.

Many first-time farmers will not get any milk out of the teat on their first try. Don't worry if this happens to you. The cause is most often an inadequate pressure at the top of the teat so the milk moves back up and into the udder instead of along the teat and into the bucket. Squeeze just a little tighter at the top of the teat and try again.

A few tries and you will have it. Your doe relaxes and you can move

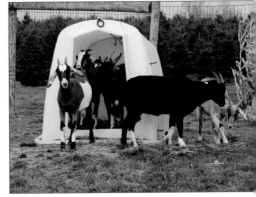

on to learning how to milk her with both hands in an alternating left-right-left-right fashion.

When the flow stops you can give a gentle bump to the udder with your hand still wrapped softly around the teat. Then tighten-squeeze-release once or twice more.

Before releasing your doe, cover and set the milk pail aside, then quickly dip and dry her teats and massage in a small amount of bag balm. You'll be hastening to the house to filter and cool the milk even if you choose not to pasteurize. Pasteurization is fully described within the dairy cow chapter.

Unpasteurized Milk

For a host of reasons some people choose not to pasteurize their milk. If you've decided this method is for you, filter the milk immediately and begin the cooling process. Don't expose the milk to sunlight or fluorescent light during the cooling process. The basic rule of thumb is that goat milk should be cooled from 101 degrees Fahrenheit (at time of collection) down to 38 degrees Fahrenheit within one hour of milking.

Never add new milk to old milk or warm milk to cooled milk.

Excess milk can be frozen in glass containers. When you need the milk, simply let it thaw in the refrigerator for twenty-four hours, shake it up, and it is ready for use. If you notice a change in flavor after freezing, use it for baking or to make cheese, butter, or soap.

Fiber Goats: Combing Cashmere and Shearing Angoras

The down-like hair that grows in small clusters under the main coat of a goat is cashmere. You will only see it if you live in a northern climate. As stated in the breed section, many breeds are capable of producing cashmere, but not many produce enough quantity to make collecting it worthwhile.

Cashmere can be obtained through shearing, but most of us with just a few goats opt to comb out the cashmere instead. Daily combing for fifteen to twenty consecutive days right before the goats' own bodies start shedding the hair in mid-December is required for the highest yields.

Save collected fibers in a cardboard box or paper bag without the long primary hairs that your comb picks up. Expect to collect anywhere between one-third and one full pound per goat.

Angora goats create enough fiber to make the process viable through shearing. An Angora goat's short fibers are mohair. The longer fibers are called kemp.

Yearlings give the finest hair and yield the highest price as their mohair is used for clothing. Shearing isn't a rite of passage—any kid with four-inch-long hair can be sheared. Adult hair is used in carpets and upholstery. The average doe, buck, or wether hair is four to six inches in length and grows approximately three-quarters of an inch per month.

Shearing of Angoras is performed just before kidding (in early spring) and then again in the fall (between weaning and being rebred for the next season). It is important not to procrastinate on the second shear of the year. Angoras need ample time to regrow their coats before the weather turns cold.

You could shear your goats yourself or hire a professional either to train you on technique or to shear your goats for you. A few days before shearing, clean out the barn, bring the goats in, and keep them dry. Wet mohair is not only difficult to remove, it is also prone to mold during storage. You do not need to wash and dry the fleece before sale, but you could net a higher price if you do.

If you have kids, shear them first on a clean workspace. Have a helper on hand to pick short hairs and any irregular, stained, or matted clumps out of the fleece. Then roll each fleece inside out and bag it individually in a cloth bag, paper bag, or cardboard box. Tag each package with the goat's name so you can record and track fleece weights from season to season. When you are finished with the kids, sweep the area clean and follow the same guidelines with the adults.

After shearing you may need to keep your goats inside for a full thirty days (the average length of time to grow three-quarters to one inch of hair) if the weather is harsh. Complications of exposure are sunburn, hypothermia, or pneumonia.

You can expect three to four pounds of the finest hair from a yearling and six to twelve pounds per shearing from an adult Angora.

Goat Meat

Gram per gram, goat meat is lower in calories, fat, saturated fats, and cholesterol when compared to beef, pork, lamb, and even to skinless chicken. (USDA National Nutrient Database for Standard Reference, Release 20, 2007)

Goat meat is also known as chevon (meat from a young, but mature, goat), cabrito or chevrette, (meat from a milk-fed kid) and chivo or mutton (meat from an older goat). The flavor and tenderness of the meat is similar to wild venison—the most coveted coming from a young animal—and can be prepared in stews, as steaks or burgers, or a dinner roast.

As you've read in the strategy section on raising goats (above), goats vary in their sizes and growth rates across the breeds and crossbreeds. You can count on fifteen pounds of freezer meat from the youngest dairy goat up to sixty-five pounds from an eight-month-old Boer.

Breeding, Kidding, and Care

Even though your doe might think she is ready to breed at six months of age, don't allow it until she is at least eight to nine months old. A better measurement is to wait until she has reached at least 80 percent of the average mature size for her breed. If bred too young, a doe's growth will be stunted, and she'll have less chance of future multiple births.

Milk goats are bred every year, usually during September and October. After a five-month-long gestation they give birth at the start of spring, when fresh pastures naturally provide the most nutrition. Meat and fiber goats are often bred every eight to nine months with the optimum breeding time between August and October. Angora goats are bred between August and November, right after a fall shearing to ensure they're ready to kid right after the spring shearing. Goats raised for cashmere are bred well before November. All kids should be weaned by mid-June, as lactation slows the growth of cashmere.

Choosing a Buck

Finding a suitable buck can be challenging. Although goats are gaining in popularity, not many people keep bucks on hand for breeding. If you keep specialty goats and want kids to keep, register, or sell for any purpose other than meat, the qualities you desire in a buck may not exist within a day's drive.

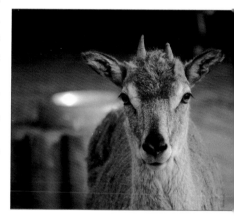

With dairy breed bucks, look for owners who keep good barn records on ancestry. A dairy breed buck will pass on the genetics of his dam if a doeling is produced. Furthermore, if your doe is polled and she breeds with a polled dairy buck the offspring will only have a 50 percent chance of fertility.

If you are only breeding to freshen a dairy doe and aren't planning on keeping the kids long-term, any healthy buck of any breed and comparable size will do.

Bucks and Breeding

A buck should be wormed and in excellent health. He should also have been on a concentrate ration for at least two months prior to breeding. Ask to see the buck's immunization and vaccination schedule. Check carefully for a CAE/CAEV clear certification.

Steer clear of bucks with poor conformation, bad legs, or improper hoof care—no matter what registration or paperwork is shown and even if you only plan on raising the kids for meat. A buck with a dull coat, very thin hair, or with patches missing may have lice, ticks, or ringworm—which will all be passed on to your doe.

A ready-to-be-bred doe will stand quietly by a buck when placed in the same area. A doe who is not ready will repeatedly move away at his every advance. A buck may mount a doe several times during breeding. Successful mating is noted by the extreme arch in the buck's back upon completion.

If you will be registering the kids, ask the buck owner for a service memo. The information you'll need for registration includes the date of breeding, the names and registration numbers of the doe and the buck, both owners' names, and the buck owner's signature.

Artificial Insemination

Artificial insemination (AI) is relatively new to goat breeders but saves the hassle of keeping a buck or transporting one goat to the other. You'll be able to pick and choose amongst hundreds of available registrations to find the exact traits required to improve your herd from one breeding to the next.

Although I have heard of some small farmers performing the insemination themselves, the process is far beyond the scope of this book. If you think AI is your best option, find a practitioner in your area and obtain a service catalog of candidates. Veterinarians are a great place to start, as are goat husbandry magazines.

A practitioner or veterinarian will assist you in locating a buck that has all the qualifications required, obtain the semen, and inseminate your doe. You may need to transport your doe to the practitioner or he may come directly to you on the date you specify.

Pre-Breeding Considerations

Before breeding your doe you'll want to put a few extra pounds on her. This fattening up before breeding is called flushing. When a doe gains weight more eggs move from her ovaries and are available for fertilization. Not only will she have a better chance of becoming pregnant, she'll also have a better chance at multiple births.

Your doe may have already stopped producing milk before she is due to be bred. If your doe is still producing milk but her body is thin, dry her off (see below) so that she can gain the necessary weight for successful breeding and gestation. A young, healthy, and strong doe can be milked right up until two months before kidding without complication.

A month before breeding, deworm her and move her to fresh pasture once twenty-four hours have passed.

Signs of Heat in Does

Most does come into a breeding cycle every twenty-one days. Not all are obvious about their desire to breed, but some of the signs might be:

- Crying, bleating, or generally being more vocal than usual
- Producing a higher milk volume right before heat, then lesser for the actual heat (a few days) with a return to normal production
- Mounting other does
- Frequent urination
- The under-tail area may darken, appear swollen, or be wet with mucus.
- Wagging or twitching the tail more often than usual

The Expectant Mother

A successfully mated doe is said to have settled, and you'll find she sleeps much more during the 150 to 160 days of gestation. New mothers and does having multiple births often kid early. A doe that is late to kid may have extra-large kids and may require assistance. Keep watch!

Two Months Before Kidding Date

Drying off a doe is most often a natural, uncomplicated process. The doe, no longer being milked twice daily, will stop producing milk and her feed will be converted into energy that serves the kids she's carrying as well as her own health.

When you decide to dry off a doe you must do it instantly—do not dry her off gradually thinking it will be easier on her. Does dried off gradually have been noted to develop fibrosis, lower milk production in later cycles, and a higher risk of mastitis. After a week of not milking her, if she looks terribly uncomfortable, you can take some of the udder pressure off. Only do this once. Although opinions vary, I don't suggest milking her completely as it may encourage milk production. Just take enough to relieve the pressure.

A gradual switch from concentrate to maintenance ration will help slow down milk production and ease the pressure as well.

One Month Before Kidding Date

At least a month previous to kidding talk to your veterinarian about a vitamin and mineral booster of A, D, E, and selenium. Make gradual changes to your doe's diet over the coming month to ensure she is receiving proper nutrition.

One Week Before Kidding Date

A week before kidding date, remove the doe from the herd, trim her backside and udder of any hair, and move her into a quiet stall where she can kid in peace and you can keep a watchful eye over her.

Here's how to tell when the kids will be born. All goats carry their kids on the right side. As the day approaches you'll be able to see and feel them moving there. Twelve hours before they're born, they'll stop moving—you can almost set your watch to it.

Other signs that kidding is imminent:

- A change in the doe's belly. As the kids move into the birth canal the roundness of her belly shifts with them.
- If she's having multiple births her tail may go up and stay up.
- She will have a mucus discharge on her backside.
- She may paw at the ground. She may repeatedly like down and stand up, never seeming comfortable in either position.
- She may be extra affectionate to her owners.

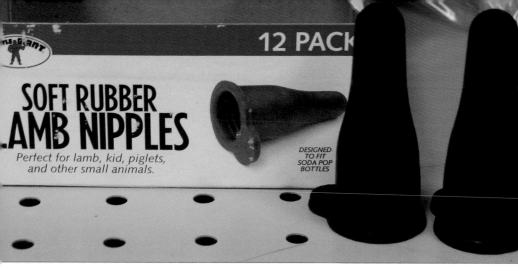

ABOVE: If you don't have a baby bottle in the house, add a lamb nipple or two to your kid kit.

Seldom do problems occur during kidding, but be prepared to assist just in case. Keep a kidding supply box at the barn ready for any last-minute emergencies that includes old but clean towels, a stack of old newspapers, a large cardboard box, iodine, a bathroom scale, and a newborn-sized baby bottle and nipple. If the temperature is still chilly add a blow dryer and a heat lamp to your supplies.

Although lamb nipples are well-sized for goats, inexpensive, and readily available at your feed store, the store isn't usually open at 2 A.M. when a doe decides to kid. A human baby bottle with an enlarged hole in the nipple works equally well in a pinch.

The kidding process usually follows in this manner:

- Doe begins to strain in a laying position.
- A water sac shows, then breaks. Two hooves appear and then a nose. A few more pushes and the kid is born.
- The doe will lick her kid and the kid will take its first breath of air into its lungs.
- A second, third, or even fourth kid may follow (dependent on breed, doe, and flushing).

Most kid births happen without interference from human keepers, but there are ways to help without being obtrusive.

Cover the wet birthing area with fresh bedding or newspapers to absorb the mess.

If the second kid is coming before the first kid is fully cared for, dry off the first kid with clean towels, paying special attention to the kid's nose and mouth. If the kid has not taken its first breath, gently tickle the inside of his nose. If the breath doesn't sound clear, lift the kid's back legs a few inches off the floor to clear mucus from air passages.

If your doe is distracted with a consequent birth and if the barn is cold, use a hair dryer (carefully) to dry the kid off. Place it in the cardboard box until the doe has finished birthing the second kid. Pull the box near a heat lamp (not too close) to ensure extra warmth is provided but only until the doe has finished kidding.

Tie off the cord with a soft string a few inches from the kid's body. Sever it at the doe's side and spray or dip the end with iodine.

Within the next twelve hours your doe will pass afterbirth and attempt to eat it. This is instinctual behavior only (to prevent predators from finding the doe and kids) and unnecessary. Wrap it up in newspapers and remove it. If the afterbirth does not fully emerge, call the vet—do not attempt to assist with this.

You can help your doe feel better after the kids have been born and are settled by providing a few tablespoons of cider vinegar or livestock molasses mixed into warm water. Ensure she has free-choice hay and fresh water as always.

How to Know If You Need Help

If complications occur during kidding you might be able to help, but if this is your first live birth, instructions from a book will be of little use. A friend or neighbor who has livestock and your veterinarian are helpful allies during your first kidding.

In any event, if your doe has been struggling for more than thirty minutes without progress, it is time to get some help no matter what hour of the day it is.

The Birth Record

If you will be keeping your does for repeated breeding over the years, record each one's gestation period and time of labor. She will be a sure bet next year to follow the same schedule—often to the same day and hour as the previous birth.

Start your barn records off right for kids you plan on keeping before you get too busy training and bonding with the new kids. Blank health dockets are at the back of this book to record vaccinations, weight, and other equally important dates and events.

Feeding Kids

The first milk a doe lets down after birth is called colostrum and it is loaded with extra nutrients and antibodies. If your doe is messy after kidding you can clean and dry her udder. As she's been dried off for the last sixty days, her teats may be blocked with a waxlike plug. You can release the plug by milking a strip from each side.

Within two hours every kid should feed. If not, assist the newborn to the teat and squirt a small amount into his mouth. He should do the rest.

Many dairy goat breeders remove kids instantly from their mother's side and bottle-feed them. This is to protect the teats, wean kids at a younger age, produce tamer adult goats, and to keep a doe's milk for household use or sale.

If your reason to bottle-feed kids is to keep the milk flowing for household use, before committing yourself to feeding every four to six hours per day, every day, consider allowing kids full-time access to their dam for the first two weeks, then splitting them up in the evening. This method allows you to milk your doe in the morning for personal use and then let her back in with her kids for the remainder of the day.

Newborn kids require feeding every few hours. By the time they are two to

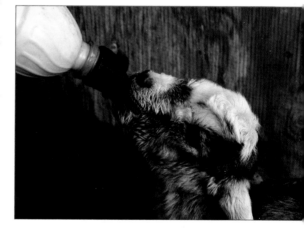

ABOVE: Many dairy goat breeders choose to bottle-feed the kids on a rigorous schedule to protect the teats of their does. This ten-pound Nubian goat has no trouble feeding from a rubber nipple and will bond more quickly to humans throughout his life as a result.

four weeks of age they only require feeding every four to six hours. Kids consume 15 to 25 percent of their own body weight daily.

After a week or so, kids will start eating a bit of hay or pasture and you can gradually introduce kid ration to their diets.

By eight weeks they should be completely weaned. The best way to decide if weaning is appropriate is to triple the kid's birth weight. When he has grown to this size, he is ready to be weaned. Although you won't need to wean fiber or meat goats (they do it naturally), you will need to wean the dairy kid. Separation from the doe for

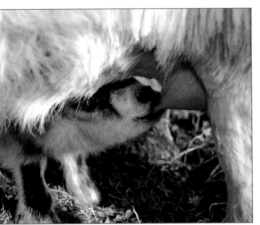

4–7 days is the norm, but once reunited watch each kid closely. If he is allowed to nurse again, separate them for another week.

Keeping Barn Records

Even if you only have one or two goats you'll want to keep a clipboard or notebook for each to record their progress, output, changes in feed, weight, and so on.

These records are valuable should you ever sell your goat or her offspring, to assist your veterinarian to determine any cause of illness, to estimate next kidding dates, and to track medications and vaccinations.

Samples of the following forms can be found in the resources section at the back to photocopy and use, or you can download preformatted 8.5 x 11-inch blanks on the Internet at KeepingFarmAnimals.com

Breeding and Birth Record: Every time you breed a doe, record the buck's name, owner and contact information, date of breeding, and notes. Attach all service memos* to this docket and record breeding dates on a doe's individual docket. Estimate kidding

---

*Service memos are available per breed registration office and are filled out and given to the doe's owner at time of breeding.

date and record, as well as date kids were born. Note descriptions, difficulties, and other pertinent information for each kid.

Barn Kid List: This form allows you to record each kid as it is born, listing the maternal doe, weight at birth, expected weaning date, polled or horned, tag or tattoo or features, disbudding requirement, and notes. You'll eventually transfer individual information to separate dockets for any animals you keep long-term.

Individual Goat Docket: Use this form to track weight, lineage, date of birth, milk production, vaccinations, ancestry, and any changes in health.

Purchase Agreement: Print and fill out this form in duplicate. One for the seller, one for the buyer.

Did You Know?

The life expectancy of a well-cared-for goat is nine to twelve years.

Castration of Bucklings

If a male kid has been born on your farm and you have decided to grow him past weaning age, you will need to castrate him. This task can be put off until anytime before puberty, but it is easier on the keeper and the buckling (as well as less risky) when performed before weaning. You can call in the veterinarian or pay an experienced local to perform the task, but the cost has the potential to nullify the economic reasons you set out to grow your own food in the first place.

The very quick castration happens at home, between the third and fourth weeks, using a lamb Elastrator—available at your feed supply store. The "operation" itself is fast and simple. By using a strong set of pliers you stretch a very strong elastic band around the scrotum of the buckling. Within a few days the testicles die off.

Feed store staff can show you how to use one, but instructions are also on the box. As always, it comes in handy to have a friend who keeps goats or sheep for first-time demonstration.

A castrated buckling is called a wether, and therefore the act of castration is known as wethering. Don't make the mistake of allowing your bucklings to mature without being wethered. The meat from a buck is distasteful and of no use. Wethers grow faster than intact bucks and won't need to be separated from your does on pasture or in the shed.

Horned or Polled

Some purebred dairy goats are born with horn buds that will grow into dangerous and difficult-to-manage horns. The polled (non-horned) trait is interestingly linked to genetic infertility. Polled bucks bred to polled does result in infertile offspring 50 percent of the time. If you need to breed a polled doe, you'll need to find a disbudded or horned buck.

Disbud any dairy kids born on your farm for the safety of herd-mates and yourself. Non-dairy breeds spending most of their time on pasture are usually left with their horns intact.

A polled goat is born with hair that lies flat where horns might have been. A kid that will eventually grow horns will have swirls of hair where the horns will appear within the next two weeks. Remove buds as soon as you see them or arrange to have someone else remove them.

I am not certain what bothers me more about the disbudding process—the bleating of the kids or knowing that I'm the one doling out the pain to such a young animal. Every time I take part in this process I swear it will be my last even though I know it will ensure a successful future for each kid.

Disbudding Kids

The technique of disbudding is to burn out (cauterize) horn buds, which prevents further growth. The inexpensive tool required is an electric disbudding iron available at most farm supply stores.

Once the iron is hot enough to mark a small piece of wood, it is held to the horn bud for fifteen seconds, then repeated on the other side.

To help ease the pain and potential for complications, trim the hair around the bud and feed each kid a baby aspirin a few minutes before the procedure. After the disbudding, hold a bag of crushed ice to the spot for thirty seconds on each side to numb the pain. If you have a spare set of hands, give each kid an injection of tetanus antitoxin (available from your feed store or veterinarian) before returning him to his mother for her own brand of consolation—a nudge at the udder. If your goat is bottle-fed, have a bottle on hand for an instant distraction.

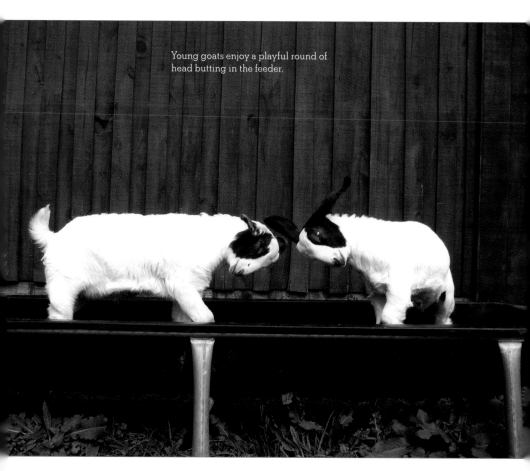

Young goats enjoy a playful round of head butting in the feeder.

Fifteen minutes later the painful memory is forgotten and kids can be seen engaging in head-butting play.

Caustic paste is an old-timers' method of removing buds. This substance is still being sold for calf disbudding, but it can cause blindness if applied incorrectly. The paste can burn through hair and skin and is better left on the shelf. Skilled herders trim the hair around the bud, apply petroleum jelly to the surrounding area, and then dab on the caustic. When used on goats, someone would need to be on hand to hold each kid for at least one half hour—while they bleat and cry and squirm to get away from their tormentors and back to momma. Without holding or confinement of the kid, the paste might shake off and burn other areas of the kid's face or other animals.

Butchering

Kids under the age of three months should be allowed water only for their last eight hours. Older kids (up to one year) should not be fed for twelve hours before butchering, and mature goats for one full day. This practice is to clean out their intestinal system and stomach, so there will be less weight to hoist over your head, less intestinal volume to clean up and out, and therefore less chance of tainting the meat.

You can employ the service of a slaughterhouse to kill and butcher your goat for you, but the economics of outside service fees may be impractical. Goats are small animals. This is one task you can perform yourself, at home.

One aspect that makes the task difficult is the requirement for room to hang and chill the carcass. Goat (and lamb) meat must age for five to seven days. If you need to take the carcass to a butcher for this, be sure to prearrange your slaughter date.

Though rudimentary instructions are provided, I would urge you to confer or work with a local, registered hunter before attempting this task on your own. Killing, cleaning, and hanging a goat follows the same protocol as for deer. You will need a rifle (a .22 is adequate), sharp knives, meat hooks and/or ropes and chains for hanging, clean running water, a large bucket, and a place to hang and chill the carcass for five to seven days (or until a butcher can accommodate you).

The kindest way to shoot a goat is to place a dish of grain on the ground. Once his head is in the down position, shoot for the spot just under the ear. When he falls, slit the throat area and immediately insert hooks or rope between the thick tendon and bone of the lower back leg. Hang at a comfortable working height and allow time for the animal to bleed out.

You must now cut off the head and tail, and all feet at the hocks. With a sharp knife and for the purpose of skinning, cut—shallowly and only into the hide—around the anus and sexual organs. Make two more shallow slits, in the inner lines of the hind legs and along the inner of the front legs. Halfway between these two shallow cuts, slit down the center from chest to belly.

Begin at the back legs and work slowly to skin the goat. You'll be pulling with one hand and gently cutting connecting tissue with the other until all the skin has been removed.

Wash off the carcass. Cut around the anus again, not deep but this time with the intention of removing it from the animal. Tie off the anus with a small piece of rope and move the bucket underneath the carcass. With a clean and sharp knife, cut lightly into the abdomen from mid-rib to pelvis, until you can reach inside and pull the anus into the body of the animal. Now pull all contents of entrails out and into the bucket, again cutting any connective tissue to release as required.

Wash out the inside of the carcass and let hang for five to seven days at temperatures of 32 to 35 degrees Fahrenheit. If you don't have available space or facility, a local butcher could finish chilling and cutting the meat for you.

Goat Milk Recipes

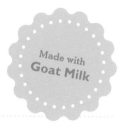

Made with
Goat Milk

Soft Cheese

1 quart filtered and chilled goat milk

½ rennet tablet (found in the pudding/
Jell-O section of your grocery store
or health food store)

1 tsp. plain yogurt

2 tbsp. water

1. Place goat milk in a double boiler and heat it to 162°F.
    Remove from heat and cool to 100°F.

2. Dissolve 1/2 of a rennet tablet in 1/8 cup of water. Pour
    the rennet water, the goat milk, and plain yogurt in a
    yogurt maker, thick pottery jug, or thermos.

3. Incubate the mixture (set the yogurt maker to 90°F or
    find a warm spot in your house at about 90°F) for 2–3
    hours until the mixture resembles curds and whey. The
    mixture will look like thick globs of yogurt in a milky
    soup.

4. Filter the mixture through coffee filters (this may take
    4–5 hours in the refrigerator).

Note: The liquid left over (whey) will make a nice ricotta cheese. You
won't have enough whey from this one-quart soft cheese recipe, but if you
increase it fourfold (using a gallon of goat milk) you'll have enough whey
on hand to make the recipe below.

Ricotta Cheese

1 quart of whey

⅛ cup of vinegar or lemon juice

1. Heat the whey to 185°F in a double boiler. Add vinegar
    slowly while stirring until whey starts to form small curds.

2. Strain the mixture through cheesecloth and refrigerate.

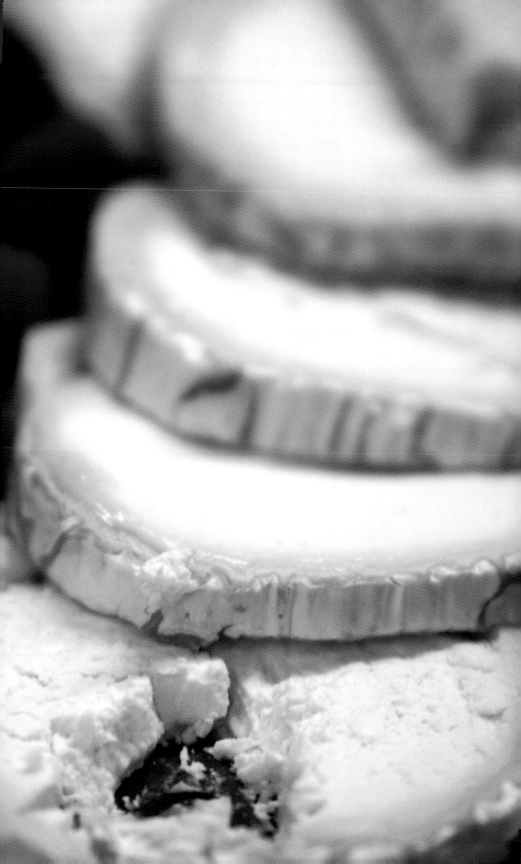

Marshmallow Fudge Treat

3 cups sugar

⅔ cup goat milk

¾ cup margarine

6 oz. chocolate chips

7 oz. marshmallow creme

1 tsp. vanilla flavoring

1. Combine sugar, milk, and margarine in saucepan.
2. Bring to a roiling boil while stirring constantly.
3. Reduce heat to medium and continue on with a gentle rolling boil for another 5 minutes.
4. Remove from heat and stir in chocolate chips until melted. Add marshmallow creme and vanilla, beating until well blended.
5. Pour into greased 9 x 13-inch pan. Cool at room temperature.

Honey and Oatmeal Soap

Have you seen goat milk soap cropping up in drug stores and gift shops lately? If you've tried it you know that it is one of the gentlest healing soaps on the market. A few years ago I gave a friend some soap I'd made during the winter months. It completely cleared up his mild eczema within 2 weeks.

12 oz. lye (available at the grocery or drug store. Use with extreme caution.)

6 cups of goat milk

5 lbs. of lard

½ cup olive oil

⅓ cup honey

1 ½ cups finely ground oatmeal (use your blender to grind it up)

1. Use stainless steel or glass pots. Use plastic or wooden spoons for stirring (do not plan on using these ever again on anything but soap making).
2. Slowly add the lye granules to cold goat milk in a large pot, stirring constantly. The milk will darken and may curdle a bit, but just keep stirring. The lye will heat the mixture up. Cool it down to 85 to 90°F. Add honey.

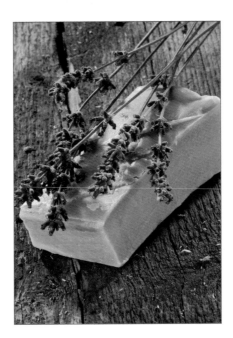

3. Heat up the lard and olive oil to match the temperature of the milk/lye mixture.

4. Slowly add the lard mixture to the lye mixture and stir continuously for 15 minutes. (If you can pick up an electric stick blender from a yard or garage sale for a few dollars it will save wear and tear on your arm. Remember though that it is best not to use it for any purpose other than soap making once you've used it with lye.)

5. At the end of the 15 minutes add in the oatmeal.

6. Let the mixture rest, checking on it and stirring thoroughly every 10 minutes until a spoonful of the mixture drizzled across the surface leaves a trail (in soap making this is called "trace").

7. Pour into molds (you can use anything plastic for a mold, even Styrofoam cups). Or put on rubber gloves and shape the slightly air-cooled mixture into soap balls.

8. If using molds, let the soap set for two days in a cool and airy location of your house. Freeze for about 3 hours and remove soap from molds.

9. Your soap will need to cure for 3–4 weeks in a cool and dry location. Turn the bars or balls every few days to allow air to cure all sides.

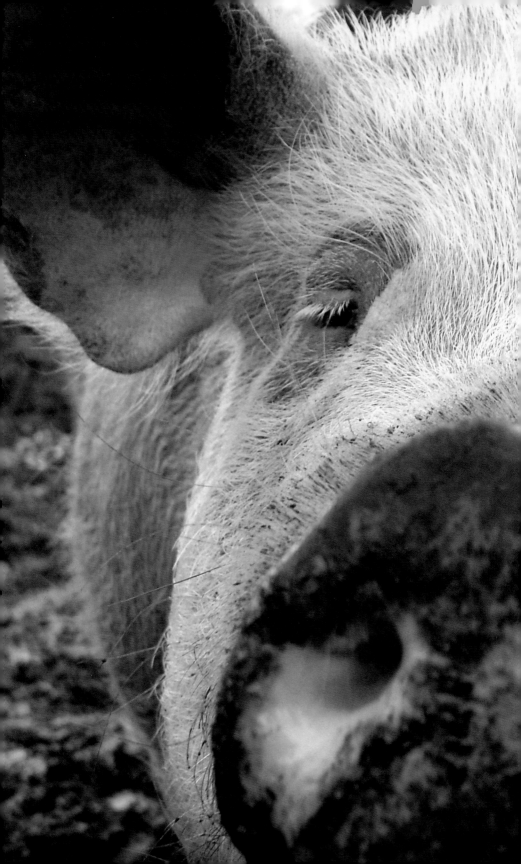

pigs

The intelligent
and sociable
pig—pet or pork?

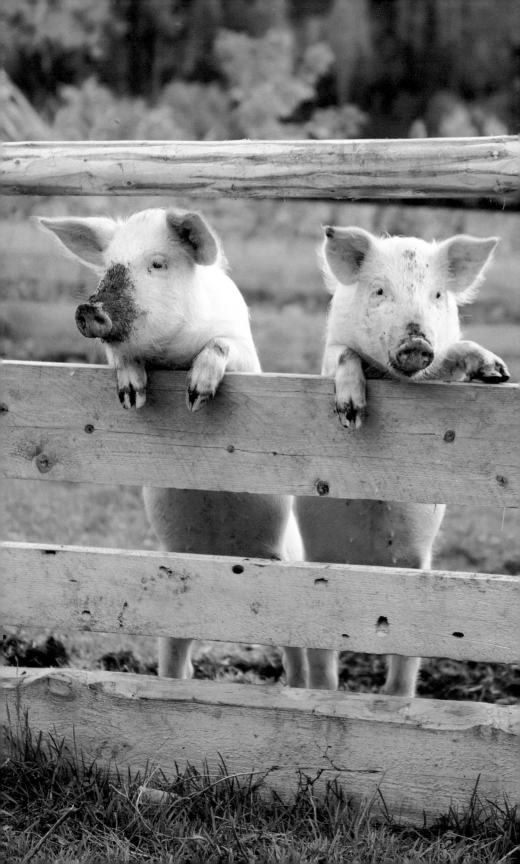

Well-cared-for pigs are quick to trust and bond with a keeper. They are unmatched by any other farm animal in this regard. They will look at you with soft and round eyes, sing while they eat the meal you've prepared, and grunt responses when you talk to them. Within minutes of passing over the barn's threshold they'll have you by the heart-strings, and in no time at all you've fallen in love with that snouty little face. Therein lie both the joy and the hardship of raising a pig for consumption.

Contrary to popular belief, a pig's preference is not to be dirty or to eat anything that lies in his path. Instead, he is a barnyard animal tidier in his habits and more par-ticular about his food supply than the vast majority of modern pedigreed dogs.

Pigs have been raised by small and large farms for centuries. They are intelligent and social animals completely capable of showing appreciation and learning simple commands. In most parts of North America, small farmers like you and I will raise a spring pig or two for a year's worth of pork, bacon, and roasts.

The pig arrives at six weeks of age when the air is just starting to warm and departs shortly after the first leaf falls off the maple tree. This is an age-old tradition built on climate, the fast growth of the pig, and temperatures cool enough to hang and chill pork.

With minimal space and bother, a pig or two could find happiness on your farm if only for a few short months. They are easier to raise than chickens if you are aptly prepared and understand their nature before you bring one home. Without this knowledge you run the risk of being outwitted by a barnyard animal, but you won't be alone. They have outwitted the best of us. Even the experienced farmer can be caught by surprise from time to time.

The Benefits of Farm-Raised Pork

Raising pork for your family's meat supply is rewarding, economical, and gainful. The finished pork excels in both flavor and texture and the versatility of the meat will satisfy even the most discerning diner in your family. Fresh, cured, or smoked; made into sausages, chops, ribs, or roasts; fried, barbecued, or braised—the possibilities of pork are limited only by your recipe books or imagination.

You'll also have an unfair advantage over the grocery store shopper. No longer will the pork on your plate be seasoned, cut, and packaged based on market demand, but by your specifications. Would you like extra pepper or garlic in your five-to-a-pack sausages? Mesquite smoked hams instead of honey glazed roasts? Half-inch-thick chops or fast fry cuts?

Far more important than flavor are the health-related benefits in avoiding commercially raised pork. News reports of mad cow disease and foot-and-mouth virus, recalls on processed meats, and similar outbreaks have left many of us wondering about the safety of any grocery store meat. Uncertainty over hormone and antibiotic residues, inhumane care of the live animal, unsanitary living conditions, and sick slaughtering practices all contribute to less than palatable meals placed on your table. No longer will those issues be of concern.

When you grow your own pork, the decisions of medicating and feeding an animal for consumption are yours to make. You can rest assured that the animal raised on your farm was given the best care and led a stress-free life. That the meat your family consumes hasn't been fed a diet of garbage, such as restaurant leftovers scraped off plates and serving dishes—some of which might be spoiled, tainted, or rancid by the time it reaches a pig's trough.

All in all, raising a pig is a satisfying and economical way to fill your health-conscious family's freezer with delicious and versatile meat. The project takes a mere five months. Daily care requires only twenty minutes, lesser still if you opt to pasture your pig.

Meat Yields for Pigs

Very little of a farm-raised pig is wasted: 75 to 80 percent of live weight will have value.

One six-week-old, 40-pound piglet plus five months of quality care equals one 220-pound pig.

One 220-pound pig butchered equals 140 to 175 pounds of fresh pork, smoked bacon, and ham roasts plus 20 pounds of lard.

The Hardship of Raising Pigs

I would be remiss if I didn't aptly warn you on this one important aspect of raising a pig. At least 80 percent of people I have spoken to, who have raised a pig at one point in their lives, have struggled over this very issue because they were not prepared.

Pigs are smart, endearing, and trusting. While they may only be on your farm for a few short months it is very easy to grow attached to such an intelligent and appreciative animal. Before you even begin setting up a pen or fencing pasture—certainly before you start shopping around for piglets—you'll need to steady both yourself and your children. Without such a steely focus, emotional scars are common.

Although it is noble to grow in fondness for the animals you keep, keeping a pig past the date you've set for his leave is neither economical nor feasible. A pig grown to maturity can easily top the scales at seven hundred pounds. He will require more food daily than a family of four and the housing or containment of such a large animal can be a nightmare. At seven hundred pounds, when you've decided you just can't keep him anymore, he will not be of optimum use to a butcher and his life will have been in vain.

For children involved in raising pigs, many of life's lessons are explored. A child under the age of six has the most potential for having her heart broken and may vow never to eat meat again. Certainly not pork.

Should emotion overpower logic and sending your first farm-raised pig off to the butcher is particularly difficult, console

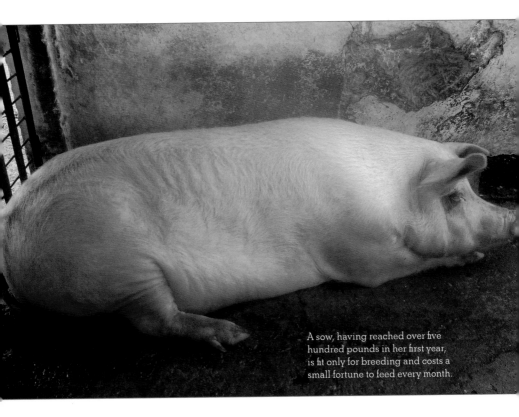

A sow, having reached over five hundred pounds in her first year, is fit only for breeding and costs a small fortune to feed every month.

yourself in the certainty that you provided a better life for the pig than a commercial grower would have on all accounts.

Deciding on a Breed

Eight main breeds of pigs are raised in North America (Yorkshire, Duroc, Hampshire, Landrace, Berkshire, Spotted, Chester White, and Poland China), but unless you are planning on raising a breeding pair, the registered and heritage breeds are of little importance. All are similar in their efficiency at feed conversion and growth rate before one year of age. Most of the piglets available for seasonal growing are purposely crossbred for feed conversion, quick growth, and resistance to stress. It has been said that these pigs grow 10 to 15 percent faster and use feed 5 to 10 percent more efficiently than a purebred.

Worry less about breed when choosing your pig and more about temperament, signs of health, overall weight, and body construction. I look for long, lean torsos in piglets and usually end up with a cross of a Yorkshire or Spot. In the past ten years many varieties and crosses have entered my farm, and each one I've raised has been as satisfying and prolific as the last.

Choosing a Good Pig

Healthy piglets have a smooth, sparse coat of hair. The skin underneath is bright and clear with no flaking or protrusions. Eyes are bright and active and noses are soft and moist or dusted with the dirt they've just been rooting in.

There is no escaping the signs of a healthy piglet when you meet one. They are alert to each other, the people at the fence gate, and their general surroundings. Any new action is investigated by curious piglets without apprehension. Young pigs who are disinterested or inactive are to be avoided at all costs.

Spring pigs, also known as weaner pigs or feeder pigs, should weigh in between thirty-five and forty pounds at six weeks of age. Any piglet weighing less than thirty pounds should be

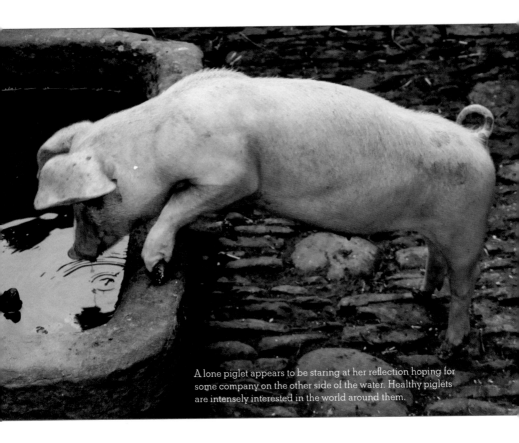

A lone piglet appears to be staring at her reflection hoping for some company on the other side of the water. Healthy piglets are intensely interested in the world around them.

overlooked—even if you have success raising this small pig he will be less economically viable.

Although good breeding practice can determine the potential of a piglet, if it hasn't had a good start it will never reach that potential. Contrary to popular children's stories of excellence in runts, a piglet abandoned by or removed from his mother before turning six weeks of age will be adversely affected in growth and health for the remainder of his life. The task of hand-raising a runt piglet is a serious undertaking not worthy of the average person's time or investment.

The castrated male pig will grow a little faster and finish ten to twenty pounds heavier than his sister. Other than this minor difference the two will be indiscernible. If you have preselected a male pig, ensure he has been castrated and the wound healed before you bring him home. Intact male piglets are not a bargain at a livestock auction. You will either need to castrate the piglet yourself or have a tough time raising him (boars can be aggressive from a very young age) as well as ending up with pork that isn't fit to eat.

Designing Your Small Farm Strategy

People who have raised pigs for years will tell you that they grow faster, larger, healthier, and happier if they have their own kind about them. I've not seen valid research on this theory, but knowing the nature of the pig, I buy into the concept every year.

If your family doesn't have a need for two butchered pigs in the freezer, buddy up with a friend or two and split the costs and chores. Even in our very small circle of friends, there are always one or two who jump at the opportunity to have farm-raised pork in their freezers come fall.

Although a pig's feed is inexpensive when compared to the amount of meat he provides, you can save between 30 and 40 percent of your feed bill by growing him on pasture. This strategy also removes the chore of waste removal and will assist you in returning any overgrown area of your farm to a pasture state. Having raised both sorts, I now prefer the pasture-raised pig. They have consistently been the happiest, friendliest pigs with the best-tasting meat.

A Pig's Temperament

A pig is an inquisitive animal with a sharp memory. Quick to figure out the operation of latches, levers, or valves, they will use their talents to create a surrounding that suits their needs. This could be as innocent as puddle creation but as devious as an escape.

A pig will also attempt to amuse himself if bored. Having another piglet to grow with or toys to play with will keep him out

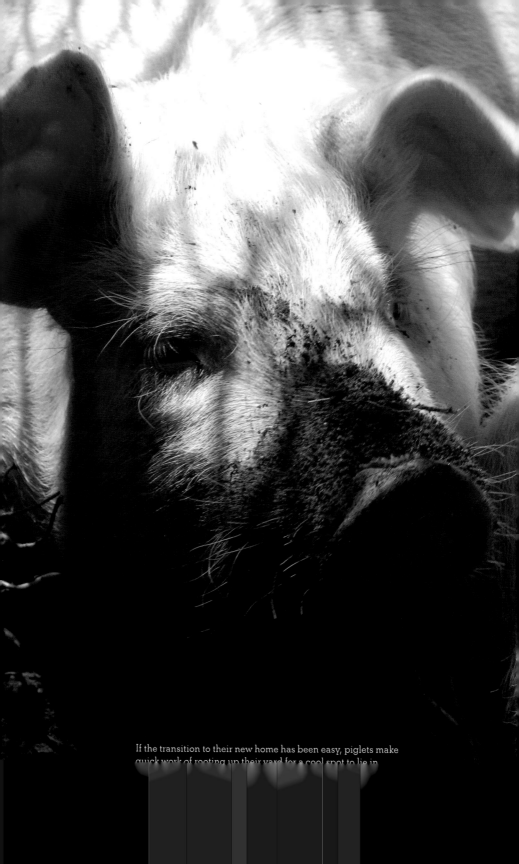

If the transition to their new home has been easy, piglets make
quick work of rooting up their yard for a cool spot to lie in.

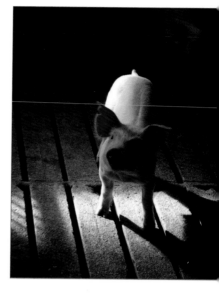

RIGHT: Pigs can be raised alone as long as they have ample company from humans or another farm animal, but in my own experience they do far better with at least one of their own to grow with.

of trouble and mentally stimulated. He'll happily push around large sturdy balls for hours in the pasture, as well as enjoying a tire swing to butt with his snout.

Although a pig can be raised individually, their very nature dictates otherwise. Pigs are social animals. It just never sits right with me to see one being raised alone in a pen at the back of the property, given no toys, company, or attention except for required twice daily visits for fresh feed and water. Yes, raising just one pig can be done successfully, but at what quality of life to the sociable pig?

Mentally Tethering a Pig to Home

When you first bring a piglet home, spend a few weeks getting to know each other in the barn or in a nearby outside pen. This gives him the opportunity to bond with family members and associate this new, safe place as home. Doing so mentally tethers the pig and is invaluable to the pastured pig farmer as well as owner of pen-raised pigs. This will be the place to which he'll return should he ever break free.

Should your pig escape, he isn't likely to go too far once he has bonded to you or to the barnyard. He will, however, get into someplace you won't want him. Flower gardens are favorites as are children's wading pools.

Call a pig back into the pen with a tempting snack and fix the fence while he eats. If he is stubborn about going back in, you can move him with a few good smacks on the butt. If he is adamant about staying put, consider staying with him to ensure he doesn't get into too much trouble. When he's sufficiently hungry or decides that he's discovered enough for one day, he'll return to the place you've prepared.

Some farmers never have any trouble with pastured pigs, pens, or fences. Could it be that they just know how to pick a good pig and build a great enclosure? Or might it be that all of a pig's needs are met within those confines and he has no desire to escape? The answer lies more within the second question. Pigs—fed and watered adequately, given a shelter that is full of soft bedding and overhead protection, provided with ample space, company, or toys to alleviate boredom, a wallowing hole to cool off in, and gentle summer breezes blowing through the area—will rarely test the fence. Would you?

Pig Pens and Pasturing

A six-week-old, fully weaned piglet will miss the warmth and security of his mother and littermates. He is optimally kept in an area that maintains a temperature of 85 to 90 degrees Fahrenheit for at least three weeks. A heat lamp or heater directed toward his bedding area is all that is required. At sixty pounds, your piglet will have grown enough to manage cooler evening temperatures of 65 to 70 degrees. Extra bedding material and a second piglet can make up for a drop of another 5 to 10 degrees.

Bedding and Temperature

Take extra precautions to keep your pig's bedding area dry and draft-free. The only exception is to allow air circulation in the shelter for older pigs being raised in a southern climate.

Bedding should be four to six inches thick. A pig likes to burrow in when he sleeps. Straw or wood shavings are acceptable materials.

Wet living conditions will make a pig sick. Always place a pig's shelter on high ground.

Outdoor Housing

Established pigs, as rough and tough as they appear, always require protection from the elements and a roof over their heads when they bed down for the night. The roof keeps heat in, and rain and sun out. Light-skinned pigs will burn without protection in summer sun. If possible, keep them near a stand of trees so they will have shade without having to be in their shelter. A wallowing hole is of great use to the light-skinned pig in hot summer months.

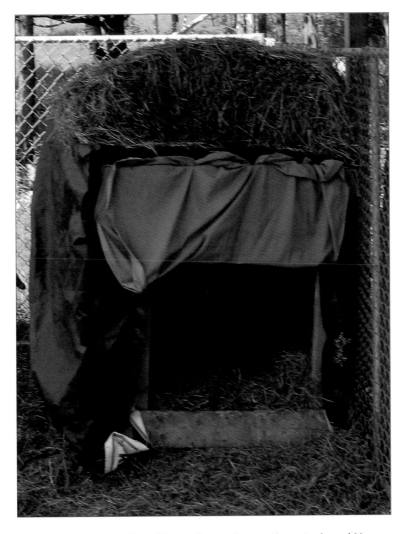

ABOVE: An inexpensive "house" for a piglet in a climate with evening lows of 80 degrees Fahrenheit. This shelter is constructed of tightly fitted 2 x 6-inch boards, tarp to deter drafts, and lots of bedding material inside. Extra bedding stored up top serves double duty as roof insulation. The height of this house is excessive, but all other structural needs have been met.

Shelters are constructed with three-foot-high walls on at least three sides and a rainproof roof.

The shelter must be large enough for the pigs to completely stretch out in. Most pigs prefer to sleep together.

Make the shelter sturdy enough to handle the pig's weight—he will be flopping around inside as well as rubbing up against the outside to scratch himself.

Bedding should be changed when soiled and kept at a minimum height of four inches when replaced. Pigs like to burrow in for the night—warm, dry, and partially covered by their bedding material.

If you build their house with a base it will be easier to move to pasture or rotational pasture.

Wallowing Zone

A pig's joy over mud holes and puddles is more about staying cool than a passion for muck. If you have the room, allot an area in their pens or pasture for a large puddle.

If you don't provide a wet zone they will attempt to make their own by spilling drinking water every time you turn your back. These highly intelligent and inquisitive animals will also figure out, in short order, how to operate automated watering devices. They'll play with valves and levers until they've created a puddle large enough to wallow in.

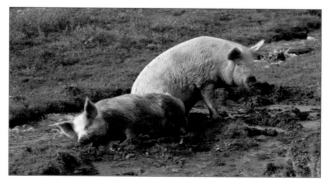

ABOVE: Pigs enjoy puddles more than they do mud, but either is welcomed as a means to cool themselves off on a hot day.

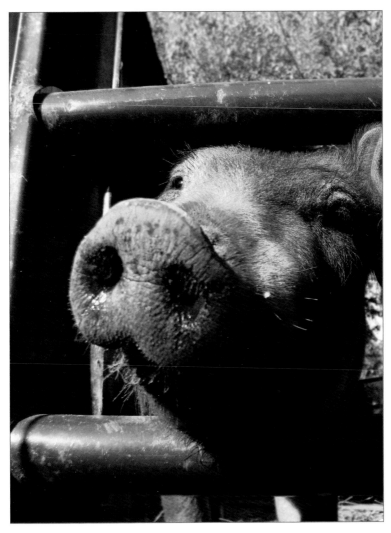

ABOVE: Heavy-duty cattle panels may work fine to contain larger pigs that have lost their interest in discovery and escape.

The Penned Pig

A pen must be, at the very least, spacious enough for a pig to change direction without bumping into the perimeter.

Well aware that a world to explore exists outside the space you have allotted for them, pigs will look for a way out. If their living conditions are inadequate or even if they are just lonely, they will even risk pain and personal safety. Once your pig has learned to knock down an enclosure, door, fence, or gate, you can count on a summer of trouble and "chase."

You'll need to fully understand a pig's ability, strengths, nature, and habits in order to contain him.

Pigs love to lean, shove their noses in, and rub their bodies on every object. Any barrier to freedom must be sturdy enough to sustain over two hundred pounds of repeated pig pressure—pushing, thumping upon with front hooves, bumping into, and rocking.

If they can't go through it, they might go under it. Soft ground at the base of a fence or gate is an invitation to root and wallow. After rooting into soft ground and pushing their noses through to the other side, they are smart enough to know that freedom and adventure are just a few inches away. Digging under the fence is less than a day's effort—worthwhile work for a pig bent on escape.

Pigs who don't feel they are getting their fair share of room, are bored, are not having their basic needs met, and have learned that fences were made to be broken will consistently test the fence.

Piglets, especially those who have not had sufficient time to bond to their keepers, will have you running to catch them more than a few times until you learn to outwit them with a pig-proof enclosure. A tightly woven wire fence works well when supported by sturdy posts, as will a four- to five-foot-high solid wood enclosure. Keep an eye on the base of any outdoor enclosure—a piglet can make short work of digging under a fence to get to freedom.

Some farmers use barbed wire in conjunction with wood fencing to contain their pigs—nasty stuff that can cut and create

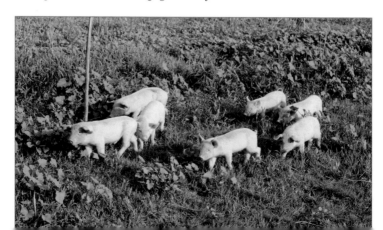

scar tissue on a young pig. Barbed wire is no longer economical in comparison to the new electric fencing units. Solar-powered units can be purchased for less than the price of ten spans of barbed wire.

Pen Chores

A pig's intelligence and tidy mannerisms make easy work of pen chores. As long their pen provides ample space they will do their part in keeping their living quarters orderly. Cleaning up food dishes, changing bedding when it is dirty or damp, and removing waste daily keep your pig clean and healthy.

It isn't a pig's preference to be dirty or to defecate near bedding or food. Allow enough space to provide for their need to keep waste away from both. You'll be shoveling out manure daily, which can be quite a chore on a hot summer day when your pigs have grown to 170 to 180 pounds. Composted pig manure is fit to use in a year's time. If you don't have a dedicated compost bin for manure, winter pig waste under a tarp and use it for an excellent show of garden flowers next spring.

I once raised pigs by penning, three at a time, in an open-roof, dirt-floor, six-hundred-square-foot barn. Their covered and walled bedding area was at one end of the long enclosure. I fed them close to their bedding area, and they used all of the extra space to charge around and wallow in a low zone I'd create with the hose. Every batch of two or three pigs throughout the years kept their waste at the opposite end, making daily removal a snap.

Inside Pens

If you will be keeping pigs inside for the duration, place them in a pen or barn stall large enough to hold them until maturity or make a plan to move them every month. The forty-pound piglet you brought home might only require twenty square feet today, but within a few months he'll tip the scales at two hundred pounds and need at least one hundred square feet to move comfortably about.

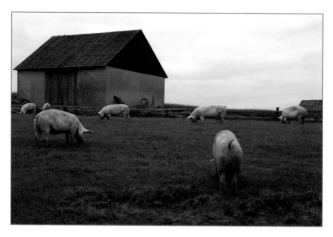

ABOVE: Pigs allowed to forage on pasture are naturally happier and grow larger, and the result is tastier meat.

Outdoor Pens

If you plan on keeping a piglet penned outdoors as soon as you bring him home, the enclosure had better be sturdy and tight. He won't yet know about electric fencing and he will have good cause to escape—he's got to get back home and find his littermates.

An outdoor pen needs to be mucked out as regularly as the indoor pen—especially so if the pen is small. As with any farm animal, more is always better when it comes to space. Although a pig can live within a one-hundred-square-foot enclosure it doesn't take much more effort to build an outdoor pen twice that size.

The Pastured Pig

Skip the hard labor of building and rebuilding enclosures, fences, and gates strong enough to hold inquisitive piglets and full-grown pigs by training them on an electric fence before setting them out to pasture.

Training a Pig on Electric Fencing

If you are pasturing pigs, you should train them young to respect an electric fence.

Within safe confinement, add one strand of live wire to their area, eight to ten inches from the ground. Keep them calm as they investigate the change in their environment. If they're charging around in a pen or enclosure they're sure to go right through the new wire, and you will have taught them that charging wire in search of new discoveries isn't such a big deal.

On the other hand, when a pig discovers electric fencing during calm investigation, one snap will send him charging back to his sleeping quarters. The pig now notes that the wire is to be avoided at all costs, although he may try it once or twice more in the next few days, just to be sure.

If you have an existing fence around the pasture, adding just one or two strands at ten inches from the ground and again at twenty inches is sufficient. If you must build a fence for your newly trained pigs, space the posts fifteen feet apart and run a strand at ten, twenty, and thirty inches from the ground.

Unlike a goat, a pig who is having his needs met will not keep testing the wire. More often than not, even if the power goes out, your pigs will remain in. Their sharp memories may lead to your dismay, however, as they will seldom cross a remembered boundary of an electric fence. To move them, even once the wire has been taken down, will take bribery or brute force. Plan your boundaries with their intelligence and instinct in mind. Don't wire gates or doorways through which you need to move regularly. If on pasture or rotational pasture, plan for their direct path home should the need arise.

Rotational Pasturing

Once pigs are trained to the electric fence, your options of where to keep them are limitless. Portable electric fencing systems allow you to move their area around your property at will.

Rotating fenced pasture has many benefits. A pig will assist in clearing overgrown land. Monthly moves to new locations ensure that they do not completely ravish any one area. Rotational pasturing also eliminates the buildup of waste and resulting odor in any one area. Nature will take care of the mess so your chore time is freed up as well.

Finally, new land is healthier for pigs. There will be less chance of parasitic infestation. As they will not be consistently running through and potentially rooting in their own muck, only to later stand in their feed trough, they are less likely to pick up bacterial infections or internal parasites. When worming medications are required, worm them a full twenty-four hours before moving them and keep them off that pasture for a full thirty days. They'll leave their infested droppings in the old location and not introduce worms into the new pasture.

When moving a pig around your land, always take his shelter to the new location. A domestic pig is a creature that thrives on familiarity. His house offers more than protection from the elements. Finally, don't fall for the belief that a stand of shady trees is sufficient cover from rain or sun, even for full-grown pigs. When his bed and housing are available he will use them.

Finding Piglets to Purchase

In the spring, keep your eyes peeled for classified advertisements in your local newspaper. You might also find a flyer at the feed store. If not, ask the store clerk for a few names of people who raise and breed pigs in the area.

When you visit a farm with the intention of purchasing a pig, you are checking for overall care and cleanliness of the barn and pens. You should hope to find a seller knowledgeable about pigs and happy to supply information such as birth date and weaned date, and have dewormed the pig the day before you take him home. He will also supply you with a few days' worth of feed so you can slowly switch your new pig over to your own preferred brand. Happily pay an extra 10 to 20 percent for a piglet whose origin you know, rather than one you may find at auction.

Many piglets are also purchased at the livestock auctions. Often these piglets are sold as full litters from one sow or a mix of runts from different sows. You'll find each in groups of five to eight.

Every so often just a pair will come into the ring at a time, which is perfect for those of us looking to raise one or two for our family meat supply.

Some nice litters have been known to appear at auction houses. If finding piglets to purchase has been a challenge and you are fortunate to find a litter of healthy piglets at auction, you'd be well advised to purchase the entire lot—even if you only want one or two! You should have no trouble reselling healthy piglets. It is often the case that even before you load too many piglets into your pickup

BELOW: Piglets selling at a livestock auction are often sold by litter. This group appears to be a good size, attentive to their surroundings, and clear of illness.

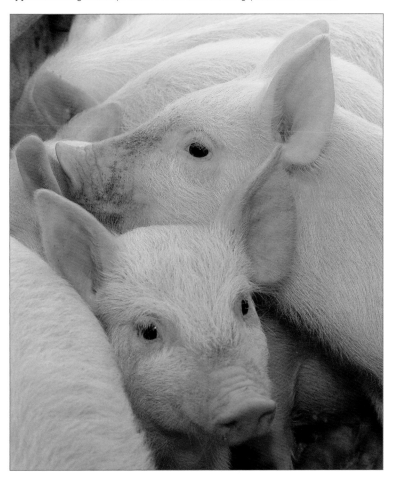

truck, you'll be approached for a sale of two or more. In that same manner, don't be shy. Ask the person who outbid you if they'd like to sell one or two of the lot. They may say no, but if they say yes your search for piglets is over.

In smaller country auctions you might be able to find out who brought the pigs in for sale. If you can, ask the seller the same questions you would have asked at the pig farm as well as the brand of feed the pig has been on. Answers to each will prove invaluable once you get the piglets home.

Should you find yourself back home from auction with more pigs than you need, write up a quick flyer or newspaper ad. You'll be down to the number you originally wanted in no time, even turning a profit in the process. Be sure to ask for more than what you paid. You had to invest the time and costs of travel, and perhaps duel in a bidding war to obtain them.

What to Feed a Pig

Not much different than you and me, a pig is healthier and grows to have more muscle than fat if he is given lots of exercise and fresh greens. This is but one of the reasons a pastured pig is healthier and tastier than a penned pig that is fed nothing but carbohydrate-laden grains all his life.

Water

Pigs overheat in temperatures rising above 80 degrees Fahrenheit. Drinking fresh, cool water keeps them from dehydration as well as heat exhaustion. During summer months, even while he's young and small, a pig can drink two to four gallons of water throughout the day.

Although there are many types of mechanical and automatic water devices available, if you're on a budget you can use any watertight, food-grade, plastic barrel sawed in half or a durable, wallmounted bucket available from the feed store.

Whichever setup you choose, you'll quickly find that a pig loves to spill, walk through, and root under it or operate valves and nipples in order to make a wallowing hole in which to cool off or play. If your system is neither automated nor secured, be prepared to make a few trips to the water daily to refill the supply.

Water should be changed daily and the bucket or trough cleaned whenever sullied. Once a week it doesn't hurt to give a mild bleach rinse to all feed dishes, buckets, and troughs.

Feed

Even pigs at pasture require a daily meal of pellets or mash to ensure their diets are complete. Penned pigs are happiest when their meals are split into two portions through the day. Commercial pig feed is the most economical and nutritionally balanced food for pigs at any age.

Recent reports on the health-related issues of commercially raised meat are based on medications and chemicals found in feed—the same feed you and I serve our home-raised pigs. Many people make the mistake of substituting corn for commercial feed as it is a natural product. Corn, however, will do little for the pig other than to put on fat. If the problems associated with medi-cated feeds are a concern, check the label at the feed store and ask for alternatives. It may take a few phone calls to find a supplier of nonmedicated feed.

Young pigs will gain one to one and a half pounds per day on commercial feed, at average ratio of 2.5:1 feed-to-muscle conversion. The average home-raised pig decreases his feed-to-meat conversion efficiency after 220 pounds.

The younger the pig, the more protein he'll require for growth and weight gain. Start your pig on a commercial starter mash that contains all the vitamins, minerals, and protein required. Then, regularly check his weight with a hog tape or by using the formula in the sidebar and switch to new feeds as set out in the table below.

Start young piglets with free-choice feeding, checked three or four times per day, until ten to twelve weeks of age, when you can

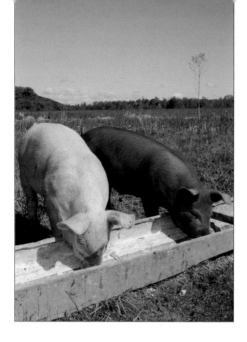

LEFT: Pigs on pasture should receive at least one meal of pig ration to round out their diets and should have fresh water accessible at all times.

switch to two feedings per day. You want to provide enough feed to ensure your pig is getting ample nourishment, but never so much that it is wasted. Spillage or spoilage, even a little a day, makes raising pigs far less economical. The table below will assist you in determining the average amount of feed required per day.

Feed Quantities and Protein Requirements for Pigs

	Pig Weight	Protein Required	Feed/Day	Consumption
Starter Grain	40 to 75 pounds	16–18 percent	3 pounds	60 pounds
Grower Grain	75 to 125 pounds	13–14 percent	5.5 pounds	140 pounds
Finisher Grain	125 to 220 pounds	12 percent	6.8 pounds	340 pounds

Weighing Pigs

Weigh your pigs using this formula: HG x HG x L / 400 = weight

HG (heart girth): Measure the pig all the way around, just behind the front legs.

L (length): Measure from the center, between the ears, to the base of the tail.

Multiply HG by HG by L and divide the total by 400.
This is your approximate live weight.
If the approximate weight you've arrived at is less than
150 pounds, add 7 pounds. If the approximate weight is over
400 pounds, subtract 10 pounds for every 25 pounds the pig
weighs.

Pigs are very susceptible to stress brought on by changing
location, being transported, and changes in feed. Limit the effects
of stress by transitioning them slowly to new feed. Over the course
of a few days, gradually mix new feed in an increasing percentage
to their previous feed.

Many farmers supplement their pigs' diet with table scraps and
garden waste. While this may be economical, as with pasture-raised
pigs, you still need to supply a commercial ration to ensure their
nutritional needs are met. I never feed a pig meat of any sort, but I
have read that many people do. Raw meat is the worst as it can carry
disease that not only could affect your pigs' health but also your
own after butchering.

An Old Farmer's Tale

When I first started raising pigs at home I was a single woman
new to living in the country but not to horror stories. I was
living on seventeen acres down a back-country road with no
friends in the area, which ultimately meant that if something
should happen to me, no one would know until the bill collec-
tors showed up!

An old farmer told me when I bought my first pigs, "Never feed
'em meat. They'll turn mean."

The thought of having two 250-pound mean pigs to manage
was enough to deter me from ever allowing any scrap of meat
to enter the trough!

Keeping Pigs Healthy

As long as your pigs arrived healthy on your farm and have been vaccinated, dewormed, and kept with care you should have no reason for concern over their health.

Keep in mind that a pig loves to eat, so if one suddenly goes off his food you can safely assume that a veterinarian call is warranted. Other signs to watch for are covered in the previous discussion of the signs of an unhealthy piglet (see Choosing a Good Pig).

Internal Parasites

Every farm animal is prone to internal parasites and worms. Pigs are no exception. Piglets are usually wormed one day to a week after weaning and before being sold. If your piglet is six to eight weeks old, it will be your responsibility to worm him twice more at thirty-day intervals.

As with all medications, take the time to read the directions and follow them to perfection. Medication residues remain in the meat tissue of a pig for quite some time. Every brand of medication differs; therefore information regarding dispersal of residue must be printed on the label of all worming medication for all animals raised for consumption.

Butchering and Preparation

You can't say I didn't warn you. For the last four to five months, you have diligently cared for this inquisitive, intelligent, and trusting animal. He likes his back scratched. He hums to you while he eats the meals you empty into his trough. In many ways he has become a pet, yes, but always a pet with a purpose.

If you've been feeding your pig finishing grain from 120 pounds on (the last six weeks or so) and he has reached a reasonable weight of at least 200 pounds, it is time to say goodbye. The finishing grain and pasture ensure that the meat will be tender, but you can further sweeten it up by feeding your pig as many autumn apples as he cares to eat. You might like to cut them into bite-sized chunks to ensure the core doesn't somehow become lodged in his throat.

If he's been on pasture, bring him in and pen him up for the last three days on your farm. For the last twenty-four hours, don't feed him, but be sure to give him ample fresh water to drink.

If you can't find it within yourself to slaughter or you are not physically strong enough to manage the task, call around to local butchers to inquire about bringing in your live pig. Some slaughterhouses also offer pickup services. For a nominal extra fee they will truck your live pig off the land. In a few weeks they will return with endless packages of butcher-wrapped meat ready for your freezer (having chilled, smoked, and cured all cuts).

I hasten to say this is not the optimum situation, as your pig will suffer some stress from being transported to a new location where the smell of death hangs in the air. However, with trusted people performing the task and your specific instruction, you can rest assured that the matter will be dealt with as acceptably as possible. You can tell a lot by the way a handler loads your pigs onto their trailer. Seldom is rough-handling necessary.

Doing It Yourself

In keeping with the farmer's creed, "If you grew it to eat it, you'd better be man enough to kill it," I'll walk you through the process of slaughtering a pig. This is tough work that requires physical muscle, so don't attempt it alone unless you know you can lift or hoist 240 pounds of dead weight over your head.

You can cure, cut, smoke, and grind the meat yourself, but that is far beyond the scope of this book. What you'll find in the next few paragraphs is the involved and humane practice of killing your pig on his own land, and preparing two sides of carcass for a butcher to further process.

First and foremost, be sure to make arrangements with the butcher for the next day. You cannot leave this point of contact for the last minute as he or she may have important information regarding government regulations that you must abide by if you employ his services. You also want to ensure that he is expecting you the morning after slaughter. The last thing you want is to show up with two sides of fresh pork in the back of your truck only to find the butcher cannot accommodate you.

The evening temperature is also important, as you'll need to hang the carcass overnight in a cool (35 to 45 degrees Fahrenheit), clean, bug-free location while you wait for the butcher shop to open. Pork does not require aging, but it must be thoroughly chilled before cutting. Your butcher will hang and finish chilling the carcass. Curing and smoking will require another week or longer.

When you go to the barn, have every item you'll need at hand. A rifle, a sharp eight- to ten-inch knife, two meat hooks (a rope or chain will do in a pinch), a strong rope or chain (to attach to the meat hooks), running water, a pulley to act as a hoist (if available and required), a few large buckets, and rubber gloves. Two people will also need three hours uninterrupted.

As I suggested in the goat section, I wouldn't suggest taking this on the first time without the help of a skilled and registered hunter. Shoot to stun the pig at point-blank range in the center of the forehead. Don't waste any time, as you may have only wounded and stunned, not killed, him. He will fall to the ground. Roll him over on his back, stretch his neck as far back as possible and make an incision through the skin and into the throat, just above the breastbone. Cut downward and in, until the blade is under the breastbone. Finally draw your knife through and straight down to sever the main artery. The pig will begin bleeding out.

Make two incisions, one on each foot, between the tendon and the bone just above the hock and hang the carcass until it has finished bleeding out. Wash off the carcass with your hose and proceed to remove the skin in strips, three inches wide at a time. This will consume most of your time on the job.

Once the pig has been skinned, cut across the back of the neck, directly behind the ears. Cut through the gullet and windpipe, then pull down on the ears, pausing to cut from the ears to the eyes and then to the point of the jawbone. This keeps jowls intact but allows you to remove the head.

Place your largest bucket under the carcass now. From the original incision, pry apart the breastbone as you cut. Be mindful not to cut deep into the abdomen or intestines. Cut around the sexual organs to within half an inch of the anus. Cut fully around the anus and tie off with a small piece of rope. The whole mess comes back into and through the abdominal cavity and out the hole you've just cut. You may need to cut a few muscles and the gullet to release it into your bucket below.

Hose out the inside of the carcass. Remove and save any large pieces of fat including the flaked leaf fat to render for lard. Finally, cut through the backbone with a knife or saw and leave the two pieces to hang and chill.

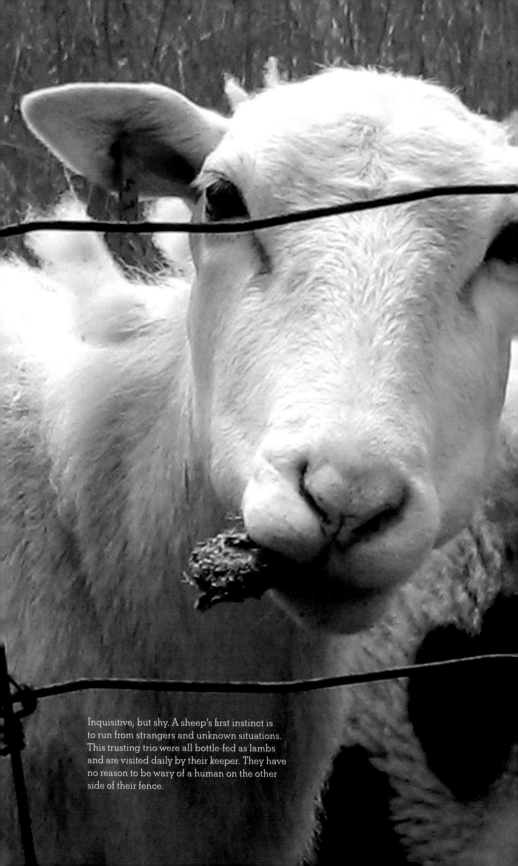

Inquisitive, but shy. A sheep's first instinct is to run from strangers and unknown situations. This trusting trio were all bottle-fed as lambs and are visited daily by their keeper. They have no reason to be wary of a human on the other side of their fence.

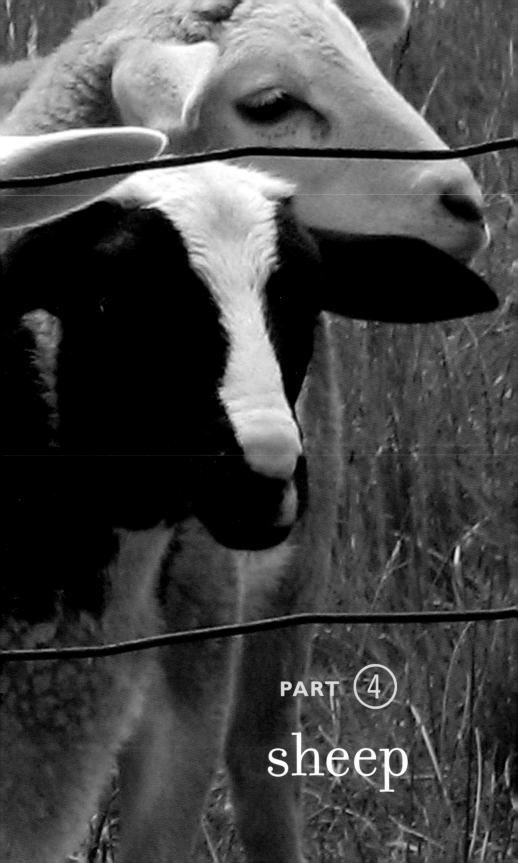

PART ④

sheep

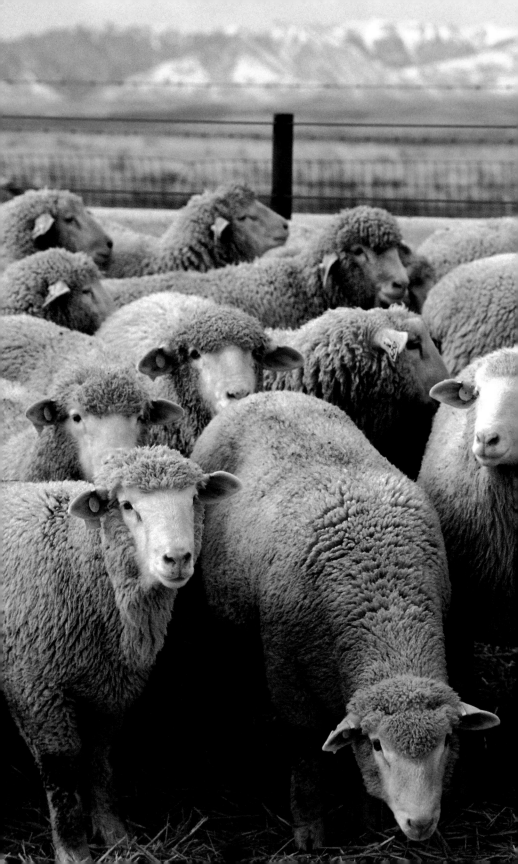

The gentle nature of sheep makes them an ideal animal for any person of any age to raise. They will grace your table with meat, provide wool to sell for an income, and create exceptional manure for gardens.

No other farm animal requires so little from a pastured field or its keeper.

Sheep are known to do well on land that doesn't seem fit for much else. If topsoil on a farm is lacking, pasture is too sparse to support cattle, or brushy growth is taking over the fields, sheep are the livestock of choice. They will make good use of the weeds, grass, brush, and even agricultural waste left over from a fall harvest.

If setting up strong fencing appeals to you more than building barns, preparation for a flock of sheep will be right up your alley. As long as there is some pasture to be had, sheep will spend most of their time outside and only require short sheds in a protected area during the worst weather and after nightfall. Six ewes and their young happily bed down for the evening in a mobile, six-foot by twenty-foot shelter, less than four feet high.

SHEEP EARN THEIR KEEP!

Sheep manure is one of the finest organic fertilizers available. It is nearly free from odor, is light and dry, and will not burn plants (young or established). Sheep manure is higher in phosphorus, nitrogen, and potassium than cow manure. If you have more than you need for your own use, selling sheep manure might be another way your sheep earn their keep!

Aside from meat that is delicious and easier to digest than beef, the wool, and the high-use manure sheep provide, they are also raised for their milk. Although sheep milk may be too much work for the small farmer and is seldom found for sale, it excels at cheese production. Having nearly twice the solids and a substantially higher percentage of butterfat than cow milk, milk from sheep can be found in some of the best European cheeses. Romano (a richer alternative to Parmesan), Roquefort, and Pecorino cheeses are three of the most popular.

Of Utmost Concern While Keeping Sheep

It is an inevitable fact of life that when raising animals for food, each one will eventually leave your farm and, while some are harder to say goodbye to than others, no amount of preparation can steady you when you lose one before its time.

This is the hardest part of keeping sheep—the morning you awake to gaze upon your peaceful pastures, only to discover the chaotic mess left behind by bloodthirsty predators. These are senseless, heartbreaking goodbyes. According to the National Agricultural Statistics Service (2004), in the United States alone predators accounted for more than one third of all sheep deaths (http://usda.mannlib.cornell.edu/usda/current/sgdl/sgdl-05-06-2005.txt).

Considering that a flock's two natural defenses are the ram (and rams are kept separate from the main flock) and running away, their ability to save their own lives in captivity is practically nonexistent. Not one of their natural defenses is a match for a band

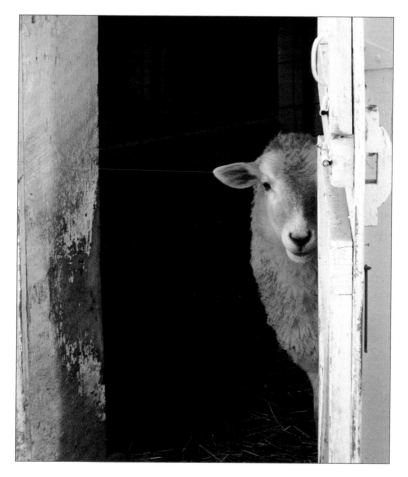

ABOVE: Having just run back to the barn (its only defense), this sheep waits at the door to see what will happen next.

of sharp-toothed and hungry coyotes, mountain lions, bobcats, or any other carnivorous wildlife in your region.

Time spent on fencing, and especially a safe night paddock, could spare you a yard of heartache and the unwarranted guilt of incompetence (honestly, it isn't your fault). Even if you live in an area where few of these predators exist, you still must keep your guard up for sheep's sake. Even a neighbor's pet dog can take a life, all in sport.

Choosing a Breed

Regional climate often dictates the breed of sheep that will work best for your farm. While some of the two hundred known breeds

BELOW: One of the more popular breeds, the Suffolk, is a large polled breed with an open face.

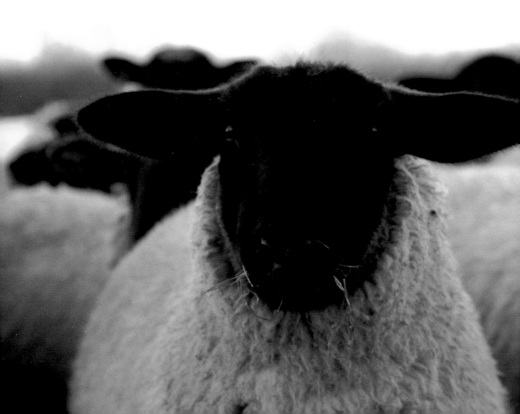

are winter tolerant, others can't take the cold. The same holds true for rainy climates versus arid.

One of the easiest ways to know which breeds thrive in your region is to take a country drive. Are there fields of sheep to which you can imagine waking up each morning and loving the view in the process? If so you'll probably find a friendly farmer tending those sheep who will be more than happy to talk about his breed. He may even sell you a few of his own or offer his assistance and advice in the future.

While all breeds are suitable for meat and wool, some breeds excel at one more than the other.

The Corriedale and Dorset breeds are excellent dual-purpose animals, as are Columbia. Columbians are better known for fleece production, but lambs grow quickly and are often sent to market at a heavier weight than other breeds of the same age. The Romney is a fine alternative to the Columbia breed if you live in a cool, humid region. The Polypay breed is the multipurpose breed of choice for meat (lambing twice per year), wool (one shearing per year), and milk production. Primary meat-purpose breeds are the Hampshire and Suffolk.

The Katahdin and Dorper breeds are also favored for meat and are an easier keep in regions where sheared wool has little value. Both of these breeds grow hair, not fleece. You may be surprised to learn that quite a few breeds of hair sheep (originating from Africa and the Caribbean) are showing up in the United States and Canada in the last ten years. Katahdins and Dorpers hold their top spots as the most popular as they are suitable for all climates, while the newly introduced breeds only thrive in southern states.

Training and Handling

Many people can't imagine that sheep can be trained. They appear to be one of the least intelligent farm animals, yet if you learn to work within their instinctual reference, you'll find they learn quickly and can be maneuvered easily—even as a herd.

With time and patience you could train your sheep to come to their name, to follow behind, and to be led by halter. The optimum time for lessons in handling is at two weeks of age, but if you use a food reward you could train older sheep as well.

A more valuable skill than having sheep that lead perfectly is learning how to herd them up quickly to move them to an alternate location. For this you will need to understand their basic instincts and work within their nature.

Herding Sheep Without Panic

A sheep's first instinct is, above all else, to stay safe by not being trapped. Their second instinct is to eat. As long as you aren't trying to trap them, and they have associated you with someone who feeds them, you can move one or many sheep to any location you desire. The trick is not to chase them. You will need to entice them to follow you.

Should you need to quickly move sheep away from trouble, keeping yourself calm will net the best results. Herd or lead them into an area they perceive as being spacious, not confining. To get them into a confined space quickly, your only safe option is to get them to follow you. They will not go, without potential for casualties and a new distrust, if chased.

Trust and Reward Training

Set aside some time to spend with your sheep and without an agenda. Keep in mind that the first step is trust, the second is reward. Work on one adult ewe or young lamb at a time by settling yourself into the pen on a short stool. Have treats of grain, peanuts, or apple wedges on hand and wait. Patiently. There are but two rules to this training exercise: (1) no sudden movements, and (2) never grab at your sheep.

Talk softly so the sheep becomes familiar with your voice while you wait. Out of curiosity, the ewe or lamb will eventually approach. When it does, should it discover the treats you have brought, let it have them. Furthermore, if every time a sheep takes a treat from you, you say its name, it learns to associate the sound of the word as a joyful trigger.

How to Handle Sheep

Sheep are quite particular about how they are handled. Remember that their first instinctual priority is never to be trapped, so you can see how grabbing at fleeces, tails, and ears might be an issue for them. They do love to be touched by those they trust and those who know how to handle them. A stroke under the chin that moves into a good chest scratch is their favorite way to be appreciated.

If you must hold or move a ewe or ram, the best way is to place one hand under the chin and one on the back of the hip. To move it, give a squeeze on the hip and steer at the neck. If you need to guide sheep often, or if you keep many sheep that will one day have a shearing date, you'll want to train them for halter use.

Halter training is best begun when a lamb is one to three months of age. Sheep halters can be found at your local feed supply store and are adjustable. Attach a short leash to the halter and with the utmost patience, never pulling, entice the lamb to follow you by using a food treat or with a helper at the back of the lamb gently nudging it forward.

Designing Your Small Farm Strategy

There are many strategies employed by small-scale farmers when raising sheep for meat or wool. Alter the number of ewes you keep to serve the needs of your family.

Purchase two bred or mature ewes and rent a ram for rebreeding every fall for 40 to 280 pounds of meat for your family freezer annually. (This is completely dependent on how many lambs each ewe produces and how long you grow the lambs.)

Since a large majority of ewes are capable of multiple births, two bred and mature ewes might yield two to six lamb kids per breeding. If you raise them just past weaning (three to four months of age or thirty-five to fifty pounds) each will provide twenty to thirty pounds of lamb meat for the freezer and the mother ewe will have done all the work. Grow those same lambs on pasture for another seven to nine months and you'll increase your freezer yield per lamb to sixty to seventy pounds.

Meat Yields for Sheep

Lamb meat and mutton account for 60 to 65 percent of the live animal's total weight.

A weaned lamb at thirty-five pounds provides twenty pounds of freezer meat.

A weaned lamb at fifty pounds yields thirty pounds of freezer meat.

A weaned, then pastured lamb at one hundred pounds yields sixty-five pounds of freezer meat.

Orphaned lambs are often offered for sale inexpensively as most farmers don't have time to bottle-feed. If you can commit to a feeding schedule of four to six times per day for the next six weeks or more, then set them to pasture, you won't need to feed and care for animals during the winter months.

Of course, if having the extra income from selling wool interests you, keeping two or more ewes (shearing in spring, then breeding in fall) and having lambs to raise for the freezer is also a smart strategy.

Preparing Pasture and Paddock

As sheep spend most of their time outdoors and protection from predators is vital, strong fencing of pasture is your top priority. Predators might be coyotes, a feral or family dog, wolves, cougars, or bears. Consider adding a donkey, llama, or trained sheepdog to your flock to aid in their protection behind the electric fence.

If you're starting from scratch (with no suitable existing fencing on your land), this may be the perfect time to plan for rotational grazing.

Rotational grazing is a managed and sequential allowance of farm animals on sectioned pasture. The practice ensures that sheep will only be eating new growth of plants and grasses growing on the land while allowing each area ample time to regrow.

The size, shape, and condition of your land, plus the maximum number of sheep you plan to keep, will dictate how you break up pasture for rotational grazing. The easiest way is to fence the entire perimeter with your strongest material and give it the most attention, then create inner barriers with portable electric fencing units.

While planning for rotational grazing, keep in mind that sheep should have open access to their safe paddock and shelter at all times.

The best fencing for sheep is a woven-wire fence reinforced with a few strands of electric wire on the outside. The woven wire keeps sheep in, while the electric helps to keep predators out. Where you need it most—to keep sheep within the confines of your land—electric fencing alone is not sufficient. In a panic, sheep herd up and run, capable of taking down an electric fence in a flash. You won't mind them taking down the portable inner fencing on 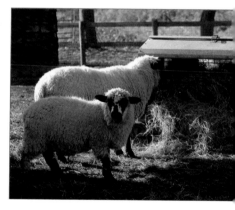 their way to safety, but if electric is all you've used for perimeters, your flock will end up at the neighbor's, in the forest, in the next county, or on the road.

Shelter from the Storm

You can easily keep sheep even if you don't have a barn. At any time of the year sheep will only need fifteen to twenty square feet each of covered shelter. It should be fully enclosed on three sides and partially enclosed on the remaining entrance side.

These small sheds need to be well ventilated and kept clean. A nice feature is that they are easily moved to clean ground within the night paddock or overturned for a quick wash inside a few times per year.

Finding Sheep to Purchase

When shopping for sheep, keep in mind that these animals need others of their kind. Even though they easily bond with humans (especially so if they were orphaned and bottle-fed) they will become miserable and depressed if left alone for extended periods. You can keep one with other livestock in the barn, but they are at their best if they have the company of at least one other sheep.

If you're just starting out with sheep, you'll be a while building connections with other sheep owners and associations in your region, but there are a number of resources to draw from. As always, a good feed supply store will give you a few leads to go on and likely has a regional sheep farmers' magazine under the counter to share. Other options are to watch the classified ads in your local news-paper or run a search online.

The increase of farming families buying and selling online in the last two years has been enormous. Try a few searches for "Katahdin Ontario sale" in Google, for example, and discover more than 20,000 results. Add your region, county, or town to the search box for more specific results.

When you visit a farm with a purchase in mind, observe the condi-tion of the sheep being raised. The entire flock should be without physical ailments, parasites, or disease. They should all have good conformation (any who do not will have been culled by six months by a responsible breeder). Over half of the herd's heads should be up and aware when you enter within ten feet of their space.

Individually and overall, look for sheep that:

- Are alert with bright and clear eyes.
- Are of normal proportion for breed and age.

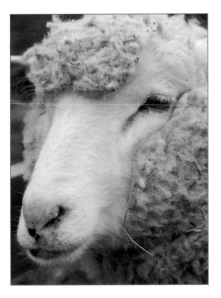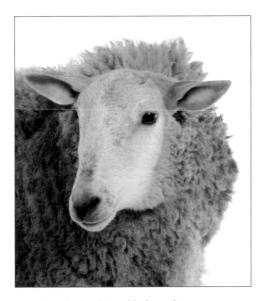

ABOVE: Closed face versus open face. Sheep are described as being black or white faced, open or closed face, prick or lop ear, and polled or horned. Polled sheep are naturally born without horns. Prick or lop ear describe how their ears sit on their head—sheep with ears that stand straight up are prick eared. Open or closed face specifies the amount of hair on the face (see photos above for an example). Some closed face sheep must be regularly trimmed to ensure wool does not cover their eyes.

- Have strong, well-muscled, and straight legs (stay away from knock-kneed, bent, or splay-footed sheep).
- Have lower jaws that are neither over nor undershot. All teeth should be present, age appropriate, and meet the dental pad of the upper jaw perfectly.
- Have a wide body with ample depth, appearing neither thin nor overweight for the breed. Watch for pot bellies, as this generally is a sign of serious worm infestation.
- Have a nice-looking fleece. Ragged, patchy fleeces are generally a sign of lice or ked infestation. Manure on the rear might be a sign of sickness or worms.

If your objective is to grow a large herd or create an income for your farm through breeding and sale of meat or wool, check ewes (that might become the foundation of your flock for years to come) for these desirable traits:

- Large bones and wide bodies.
- Normal docked tail length (although this may appear to be a cosmetic concern, a ewe with a too-short tail may have trouble lambing).
- No lumps in, or damage to, udder.
- An ancestry of twin and triplet production. A ewe that was a twin at birth is more likely to lamb multiples.

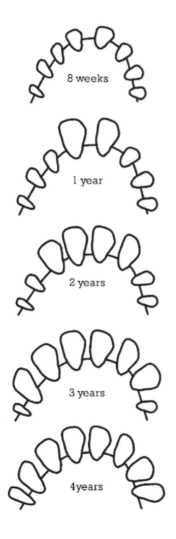

8 weeks

1 year

2 years

3 years

4years

Knowing the ancestry of your ewe is as important for undesirable traits as well. Ask the owner if the ewe had been orphaned and if so, the reason why. If her dam was not interested in raising young and orphaned her lambs, your potential ewe may have inherited the trait. It all adds up to more chores down the road. You might find yourself bottle-feeding every one of her offspring for as long as you choose to breed her.

Rams should have all the fine qualities of a ewe (other than the udder and concerns over short tails). Consult with a veterinarian for fertility feasibility before purchase.

LEFT: At three weeks of age a lamb will begin to grow baby teeth on the bottom. Sheep do not have upper teeth. Instead they have a hard upper gum called a dental pad. Teeth grow in as pairs and within a few weeks all eight baby teeth are present. At one year old a lamb begins replacing these with permanent teeth, which grow in at the rate of two per year until the sheep is four years old and has replaced all baby teeth with permanent.

Bringing New Sheep Home

Optimally, any sheep you buy will come with a health maintenance sheet and/or growth records. If the owner doesn't keep records, start your own by bringing a blank on day of sale. Before you make the exchange of cash for sheep, ask appropriate questions to fill out the form as much as possible.

All sheep, even if they are the first on your farm, should be quarantined for seven to ten days. This gives you time to get to know each other, change their feed over to your own preferred brand, and worm them if they had not been before they left the previous farm. Allow a full twenty-four hours after worming medication has been given before setting sheep out to pasture.

Feeding Your Sheep

Sheep, like goats, are classified as ruminants. They have a similar four-part stomach that allows them to graze on and digest green pasture as well as brush, leaves, grain, and straw, among many other feeds.

As they can eat such a wide variety of feeds and are curious about their surroundings, they are not aptly capable of discerning a good plant from a toxic one.

Some of the most common plants growing in North America poisonous to sheep are wild lupine, yew, oak and acorns, tomato and potato, milkweed, ragweed, sheep laurel, and nightshade. Err on the side of caution before you set sheep out to new pasture. Ask local authorities about known toxic plants in your region and familiarize yourself with each one. Walk your pasture regularly and uproot any suspicious new growth.

Feeding Requirements

All that is required to keep most sheep healthy is pasture grass while it is growing, plus a salt and mineral supplement. As pasture dies with the seasons, you'll need to supply free-choice hay.

Salt and mineral/vitamin supplements for sheep are sold in granular form. These may be left in their night paddock as free-choice. They'll take only what they require. If your feed store is out of sheep salt and vitamins, it is better to have none and wait than to have salt blocks or mineral supplements intended for cattle.

Sheep do not need grain if they are thriving on pasture and good quality hay. Grain is given as a treat, to complement poor pasture, to increase energy, for weight gain, or to flush a ewe before breeding. If you will be giving your sheep grain for any of those reasons, do so individually and gradually. Even breeding ewes being flushed require only a small amount of grain for just a few weeks (see page 177).

You may need selenium supplementation—especially if your ewe has been bred. Selenium is a trace element that has been depleted from the soil in many regions of the United States and Canada. To find out if this is a problem in your area, collaborate with local sheep farmers, a veterinarian, or your feed supplier. (If locals are supplementing other livestock with selenium, your sheep are most likely in need.)

Hay

Healthy sheep will not eat more hay than they require or grow fat by having too much. When the pasture is looking sparse or has been covered by a blanket of snow, keep free-choice hay out for them. Keep the hay accessible well into spring, as a belly full of fresh pasture, after months of being fed hay, could upset their digestive process.

Sheep will do best on hay that has a high percentage of grass or alfalfa. Avoid clover in hay and on pasture for ewes that you might be breeding as it decreases fertility.

Water

Sheep on lush, green pasture may not drink as much as they will when surviving on hay alone, but they are apt to drink more in the long, hot days of summer. No matter what the temperature, fresh, clean water needs to be accessible at all times.

Sheep will drink out of a communal, shallow water basin or trough. Ensure that it is safe for, and accessible to, lambs. Lambs have been known to drown in larger, deeper tubs. All troughs, tubs, or basins should be cleaned with a mild bleach rinse weekly to decrease exposure to bacteria.

If winter lows drop below freezing in your area, add an inexpensive deicer to their water supply or plan to visit the barn regularly to top up buckets.

A Change in Pasture

As with any animal transported from one farm to another, an immediate change in feed can jeopardize the health of the animal. Before bringing a lamb, ram, or ewe home, compare the content and growth of your own pasture with the previous home's pasture. If your pasture is lush and the sheep is used to brush and sparseness, she may need to be introduced slowly to your fields. Also if any supplements are being given, find out the schedule and the brand from the seller.

Changes in Feed

All sheep have sensitive digestive systems that can be upset by a change in feed. Any change should be made over the course of a week by slowly introducing the new food—whether it be a change in quantity, supplier, or quality.

This understanding is extended for a change in ownership as well. Sheep and lambs moving to a new herd will have enough stress to manage without adding a change in food source as well.

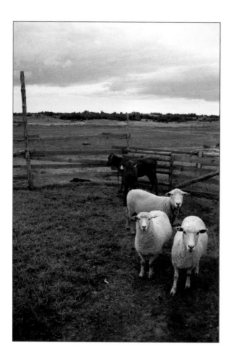

LEFT: Sheep and cattle can be raised together without complications.

Health and Grooming

The care of sheep is relatively easy. They are resilient to disease and infections as long as you are watchful of their condition and keep their paddock, water, and shelters relatively clean. Grooming chores are minimal but necessary to maintain the health of the flock.

Castration and Tail Docking

If a ram lamb has been born on your farm and your goal is to raise him past weaning for your own meat supply, castrate him to keep the meat tasting sweet. The tool (Elastrator) and process discussed for castration of goat kids are also used for both docking lambs' tails and castrating ram lambs.

RISING MARKET TREND

If you are planning on selling off a ram lamb, check current market trends before you dock and castrate. A current trend and uprising demand in many regions of the Unites States and Canada exists for unaltered ram lamb meat. Don't grow an unaltered ram lamb, though, unless you have a verified buyer.

The task of castration will be easier on yourself and on the young lamb if you castrate as soon as both testicles have dropped into the scrotum. Start checking your ram lambs daily between ten and fourteen days of age.

All lambs—even those you'll raise for just a short time—should have their tails docked. Tails are breeding grounds for bacteria, flies, and maggots. Attend to this task earlier rather than later. It hurts lambs less to have their tails docked between two and seven days of age. Lambs that you are planning on keeping for breeding later have more specific reasons for a dock—namely the facilitation of breeding, lambing, and shearing.

Diseases and Infections

Abscess

A bacterial infection on the skin of sheep, most commonly introduced through scratches and wounds after shearing. Severe cases may affect the lymph nodes.

Prevention: Check any new sheep being introduced to the herd during quarantine period. Disinfect all shearing equipment regularly and immediately treat any wounds.

Treatment: Surgery is the only known treatment although it is both expensive and not always corrective.

Copper Toxicity

Although sheep need a small amount of copper, too much can kill them. Excess copper will result in liver damage and the breakdown of red blood cells.

Prevention: Ensure your salt and mineral supplement does not include copper and only use feed and supplements made for sheep.

Treatment: As warning signs are hard to spot, there is no known treatment.

Enterotoxemia

Classified as a life-threatening bacterial infection also known as overeating disease.

Prevention: Part of your vaccination schedule.

Treatment: None.

Orf

Also known as sore mouth, scabby mouth, contagious pustular dermatitis, and ecthyma. This viral condition causes thick scabby sores on the lips and mouths of lambs that can last up to four weeks. Pay special attention to young lambs, as they may have trouble nursing and suffer from dehydration and malnutrition.

Human handlers should always wear plastic gloves when feeding or caring for lambs with orf.

Prevention: There is nothing you can do to prevent this virus.

Treatment: Clears up on its own in one to four weeks. An after-infection, veterinarian-supervised vaccine is now available to prevent further incidences.

Pneumonia

Two types of pneumonia are common with sheep. The first is a bacterial pneumonia suffered by lambs and the second is a progressive (over months or years) pneumonia in adult sheep. A less common condition of pneumonia—caused by inhalation of feed or medications—can affect both lambs and mature sheep.

Prevention: Purchase only healthy animals from reputable farmers. Keep a lamb's living quarters clean and be extra careful if bottle-feeding to ensure the milk isn't inhaled.

Treatment: Lambs with bacterial and inhalation pneumonia may be treated with antibiotics but the progressive pneumonia has no known cure.

Scrapie

Scrapie is a highly infectious neurological disease that has been likened to mad cow disease. Infected sheep will lose condition quickly and will be noted staggering, trembling, and repeatedly scraping their bodies against solid objects.

Contact your veterinarian immediately and keep visitors off your farm until you receive results from testing.

Deworming

All sheep, even lambs, need to be treated for worms under veterinary supervision, at least twice per year. You will need to worm your entire flock more often if their pasture is small or if you are not employing rotational pasture grazing.

Worm lambs between two and three months of age, and watch their growth for signs of serious infestation, which include pot belly, scruffy coat, loose manure, and prominent hip bones. Ewes need to be wormed before breeding, again before lambing, and finally before being set out to pasture. Rams are most often wormed before

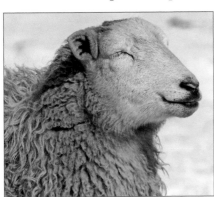

breeding and again before being set on pasture. Mature sheep may show signs of infestation with a swelling under their chins called bottle jaw.

Vaccinations

Disease and vaccinations that prevent or deter disease may be regional. Vaccinations are recommended across all of North Amer-ica for enterotoxemia, pneumonia, and clostridial diseases. Other vaccinations may be required or recommended for your region. Your veterinarian will help you determine a vaccination schedule for your sheep—including ewes and upcoming lambs.

Hooves

Domestic sheep have ancestors that once wandered rocky hillsides where hooves would be trimmed with every step. Today's sheep, wandering farmers' fields of soft green pasture, require hoof trimming as part of their basic care.

Sheep with overgrown hooves have trouble walking, may graze on their knees, and are prone to hoof disease. As every sheep's hooves grow at a different rate it is good management to check regularly for signs of overgrowth. Smaller, more frequent trims are easier to manage than a biannual trimming and keep your sheep's hooves neat and healthy.

If you will be shearing sheep, a spring hoof trim fits in perfectly with the day's work. With gloves on and hoof shears in hand, set sheep on their rumps and prop them up against a helper's legs.

Be mindful and give all the attention to the task at hand. Freshly cut hooves are sharp. While trimming hooves (follow the instruction provided for goats on page 96) check your sheep for hoof rot, plugged toe glands, foot scald, and any abnormality in growth.

Foot scald and hoof rot are most common after extended pasturing on wet land. Even though these are both bacterial infections, only hoof rot is contagious and requires veterinary supervised care. Foot scald occurs on the skin between the toes and is cured after a normal trim followed by a topical treatment and foot baths. Move your herd to drier land.

Hoof rot can be introduced to a herd from a carrier animal that may not show signs of the infection. Hoof rot occurs on the hoof itself and requires veterinarian assistance, a standard trim, and topical treatment of all sheep in the flock. Follow up treatment with the same care every three weeks until no evidence of infection is present. Sheep showing signs of hoof rot infection should receive a penicillin or tetracycline injection.

Plugged toe glands are a painful affliction that, if left untreated, could cause lameness. The toe gland on a sheep's foot can be found directly between the toes on the top of the hoof. The cause of the plug is wet pastures. Unplug the gland by applying gentle pressure to the area and follow up by disinfecting with hydrogen peroxide immediately.

Shearing Sheep

The act of shearing sheep is performed once a year in the spring. Not only will shearing make your sheep more comfortable in the coming heat of the summer and keep them free of lice and keds, the fleece can also be sold to provide extra income for your farm. Good quality fleece is a result of optimum health and will net a higher selling price.

Many small farmers raising sheep just for meat won't shear for sale, but for care. Finding little monetary gain in the fleeces for all the trouble of keeping sheep clean, the thick woolly coats are sent straight to the garbage bin. If this is your planned strategy you can save the cost of hiring a professional and shear your own sheep. Should you hope to sell the fleece, you could take a class to learn how or learn by assisting a professional shearer.

Most shearers won't come to your farm unless you have a hundred sheep or more to shear, but you could buddy up with another local farmer to make his visit worthwhile. You will be expected to prepare the area and assist in the shearing by catching and leading each sheep to the shearing floor, sweeping the area after every animal, and skirting your own fleece.

Shearing season is also an excellent time to check and trim hooves, deworm and delouse, vaccinate if required, investigate teeth, and spray with a bug repellent before releasing sheep into the paddock.

Preparation for shearing day includes:

- Keeping sheep inside for a day or two if rain is expected
- Having them all in a pen for easy catching and leading
- Setting up a shearing floor (usually a clean sheet of plywood) and a skirting table

- Checking the barn's first aid kit for iodine, adhesive bandages, and hydrogen peroxide

A skirting table is commonly a slat top table wide enough to hold a full-sized fleece. As the shearer hands you a fleece, lay it shear side down and skirt it by trimming on the natural curves. Roll it up, shear side on the outside, and place it into a labeled cardboard box.

Breeding, Lambing, and Care

If you have opted to rent the services of a ram and you have a choice among a few, choose the ram with the most experienced owner. He will know the best time for both the ram and the region. Breeding

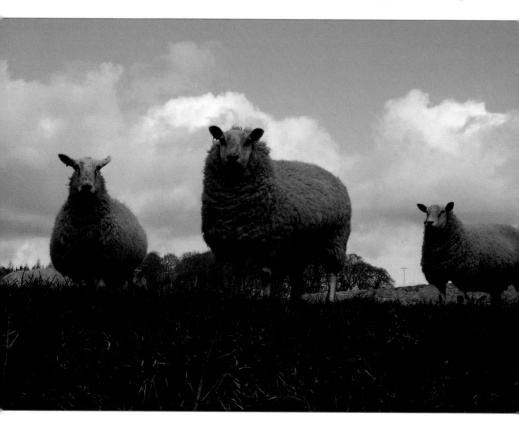

rams have specific needs in their care, the most important of which is seasonal temperature.

The gestation period of a ewe is approximately five months (between 147 and 153 days). Breed in late summer to fall to ensure that lambs can be weaned around the time fresh green pastures appear. Breeding management is region-specific and in some cases, breed-specific. The Polypay breed, for example, breeds and lambs twice per year.

Three weeks before breeding a ewe, flush her by feeding her grain to improve fertility. Start at one quarter pound per day and steadily increase her intake to a full pound per day for the first week. Carry on feeding her one pound per day for two weeks, breed her, and then gradually decrease her portion over the week following breeding.

In her fourth month of pregnancy begin giving her grain again, this time increasing her portion to one and a half to two pounds per day over the course of ten to fourteen days. This strategy ensures she's receiving enough nutrition to feed the growing lambs she's carrying without making her fat. Younger ewes may require more grain as their own bodies are still growing.

In the last two weeks of pregnancy, keep a watchful eye on your ewe. Any sign of illness, change in temperament, or lack of interest in hay or feed is a warning that something is wrong. All are worthy of a call to the veterinarian. In the last week of gestation, shear her udder and rear end if she is a wool breed or has manure buildup.

Lambing Day

Although lambs are usually born on pasture, they are best kept in the barn or a shed for their first few days where they can bond with their mothers. Keeping them confined also keeps them out of cool drafts or being accidentally trampled by inquisitive ewes. In the barn you can watch over and ensure that they are feeding and that all is well before releasing both ewe and lamb back onto pasture.

For the purpose of containing ewe and lamb, construct four-foot by six-foot temporary stalls (also known as jugs) in a barn or shed, and then remove them and set them aside for another year. A standard jug is three feet high. Jugs can be made of plywood to assure that drafts will not affect the newborn lambs, but many sheep farmers with draft-free enclosures use slatted skids. Jugs are best constructed to allow for easy adjustment. A ewe with triplets would be far more comfortable in a six-foot by six-foot space, while sick, injured, or orphaned lambs only need a four-foot by four-foot space.

Jugs are only used after the lamb has been born. An expectant ewe will resent being penned up before birthing, as moving around, lying down and standing up, pawing at the ground, and finding her own place to birth are part of a ewe's delivery process and her rite of passage.

More often than not the act of lambing is carried out without human assistance. The processes of lambing and kidding (birthing goats) are similar, from the signs of imminent labor to care of the newborn; see "The Expectant Mother" in the Breeding section of the Goats chapter starting on page 107.

Once the lamb has been born and his face is clear, he is breathing, and he has been licked and accepted by the ewe, everything should be fine. If these conditions have not been met within ten to fifteen minutes, you can partially assist by clearing the lamb's face, rubbing him briskly with towels to stimulate breathing, and placing him by the ewe's head.

Once she has accepted her lamb and as long as the temperature, weather, or barn floor conditions are acceptable, you can allow her a half hour of uninterrupted time before moving her and her lamb to their private jug. Carry the lamb slowly, so she can see you and hear the lamb, and she will follow.

In the jug you can care for the lamb by snipping the umbilical cord (two inches away from his body) and dipping what is left on his body into a tamed iodine solution. Give your ewe a drink of lukewarm water with a tablespoon of molasses mixed in. While she's drinking, ensure her teats are open by squirting just a little from each one. Teats may have plugged since the last lamb was weaned eight months ago and will open up with a gentle squeeze.

By the time you have moved them to the jug, the lamb should be able to stand and should want to nurse. If there are complications you may need to assist, even by the most intrusive act of milking the ewe and feeding the lamb by baby bottle. A standard newborn child's bottle works best, earlier softened by previous use or boiling water, and with an enlarged hole in the nipple.

The first few ounces of milk contain the most important nutrients from the ewe. Colostrum (first milk) carries natural antibodies, minerals, and laxatives to get the lamb started off on a path to a lifetime of good health.

Should the ewe reject her lamb altogether you will need to continue feeding the lamb by bottle on a schedule of four to six times per day for the next six weeks. Allow the ewe and lamb at least a day to bond in the jug before committing to full-time

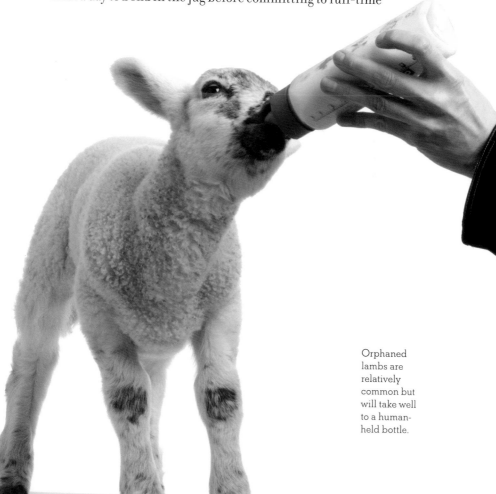

Orphaned lambs are relatively common but will take well to a human-held bottle.

bottle feeding. During the first twenty-four hours, if you have not seen the lamb nursing every few hours, keep bringing the lamb a bottle of sheep milk or sheep milk replacer.

While you keep ewe and lamb(s) in the jug, do not feed the ewe grain but allow free-choice hay and fresh water as always. Water buckets should be small and topped up regularly. Once you release them both you can increase her grain ration again to one and a half to two pounds daily—split into two servings throughout the day—as she'll require more energy to make milk for her lamb. Begin reducing the ewe's grain again three weeks previous to weaning.

A ewe's milk supply or desire to nurse will dictate the age of weaning. This occurs between three and four months after the birth. If you plan to keep the milk for personal use (such as to make cheese), you can rush the weaning date by a few weeks by separating the two during the day and allowing them to be together during the night.

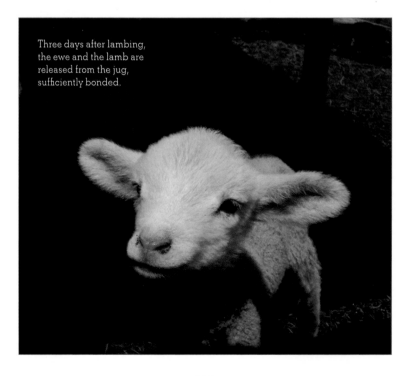

Three days after lambing, the ewe and the lamb are released from the jug, sufficiently bonded.

Feeding Lambs

Sometime in the second week of their lives, lambs will begin nibbling at pasture and hay by their mother's example and may show an interest in her grain.

To ensure lambs receive necessary feed for growth and health, construct a creep feeder of wire or wood that allows free-choice entry for lambs, but keeps larger ewes out. The standard size of entry for lambs is fifteen by eight inches. The area inside should contain a manger of hay, a supplement feeder, fresh water, and clean bedding on the floor.

Butchering

As lambs and adult sheep are small, you can certainly slaughter and butcher them yourself at home. The carcass will need to be hung and aged for seven to ten days in a 30- to 35-degrees-Fahrenheit protected space before being cut into chops and roasts. As most small flock owners don't own a walk-in freezer, they put off butchering until the weather turns cold enough and hang the carcass in a shed, or they employ the services of a butcher for hanging and wrapping.

The method of slaughtering sheep is the exact same as the one used for goats. Please see the Butchering section in the Goats chapter on page 117 for a complete description.

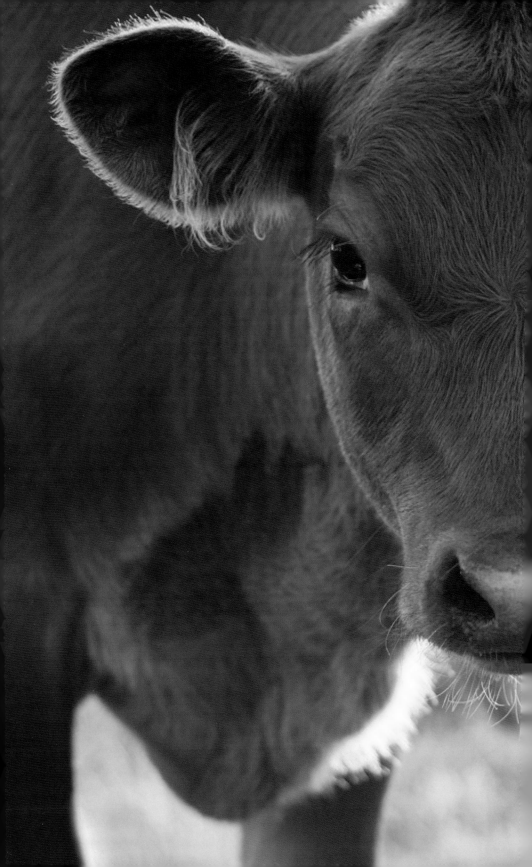

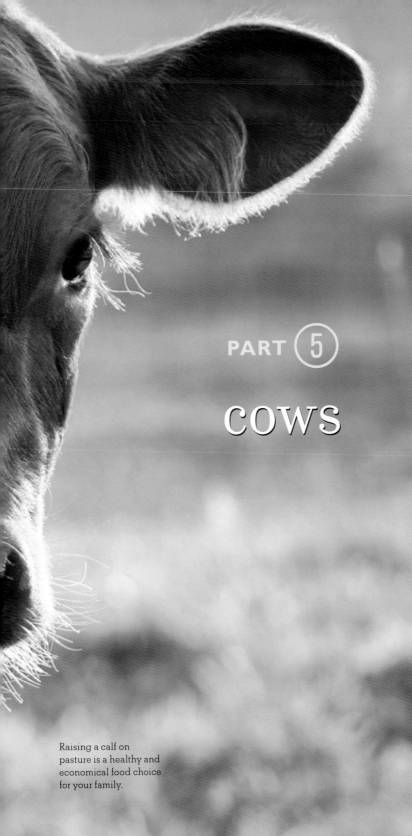

PART ⑤

COWS

Raising a calf on
pasture is a healthy and
economical food choice
for your family.

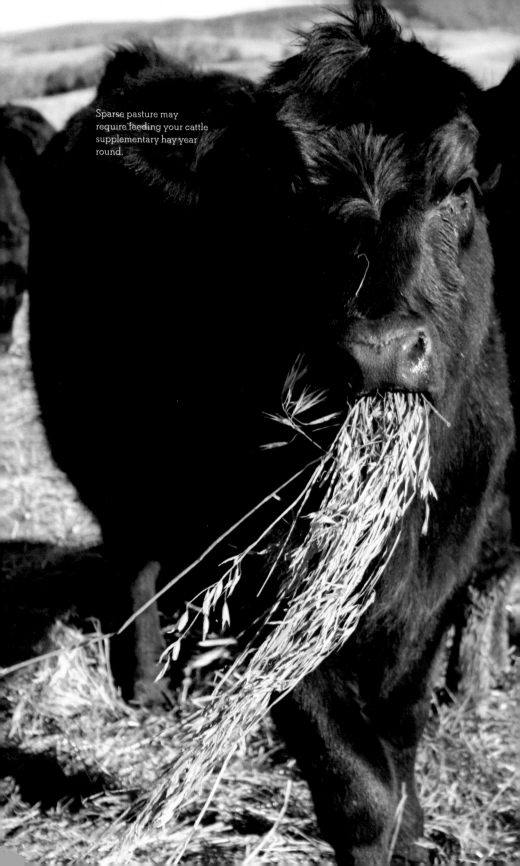

Sparse pasture may require feeding your cattle supplementary hay year round.

In the old days every homestead with a family to raise had at least one cow on pasture or in the barn. To the farmer who kept her she'd supply a source of milk for nine to ten months of the year and enough beef to feed the family throughout the next year by her offspring.

Her milk was fed fresh at the table or made into cheeses, yogurt, ice cream, and treats, plus any surplus helped to sustain pets or her barnyard companions. The beef of her young, raised nearly without cost on pasture until the snow fell, was higher in vitamins and nutrients than today's grocery store beef, even with all of our modern-day advances in science and animal husbandry.

The reason modern beef pales in comparison is all in how it is raised. Beef that shows up in your grocery store is more often than not the product of cattle finished on a diet of grain in a feedlot. A lot of grain in fact. And for many months.

On the surface this doesn't sound odd. After all, grain increases bulk and marbling within the muscle of cattle. With all that extra fat throughout, the beef is juicy and delicious. But the problem is that cattle digestive systems were not meant to survive solely, or even mostly, on grain. In fact, all that grain makes cattle sick, causes liver dysfunction, and stresses their immune systems.

Feedlots counteract cattle's reluctance to consume so much grain by giving them hormone shots that increase their appetites. Now the cattle will eat almost anything. You can research precisely what "almost anything" is online or through recent documentaries. I promise you'll never touch a grocery store steak or a fast-food

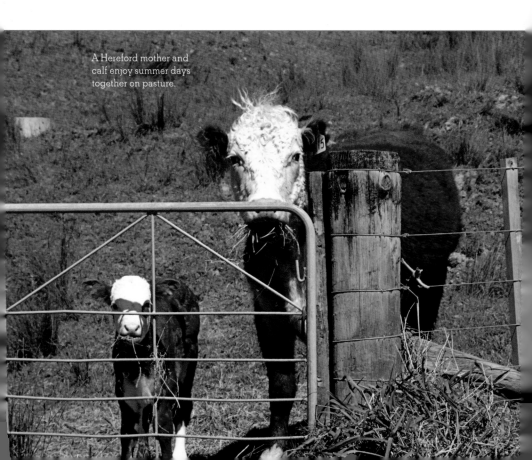

A Hereford mother and calf enjoy summer days together on pasture.

burger again. The cattle, sickened by the feed they cannot help but eat, are then given medications to fight infections and override liver, organ, and system failures. Sicker still and loaded with chemicals, hormones, and antibiotics, the cattle's discomfort becomes an acceptable norm. Acceptable to the feedlot owners, perhaps, but not to the cattle.

One day, this has to stop. This is why I applaud every person on a mission to raise his or her own food. Not to upset the balance of corporations profiting from pain—after all, not all feedlots are created equal—but to reinforce your ideals with one more reason to carry through.

Healthy milk and beef aside, the purest joy of raising your own cattle is that you do not need to cause suffering in the final days of an animal to feed your family. Pasture-raised beef is equally as tasty as the feedlot variety and, as an added benefit, is one-third to three times leaner than grain-fed beef.

Here's more great news. Beef raised on pasture has two to four times more cancer-fighting omega-3 fatty acids, plus more vitamin E, beta carotene, and folic acids than grain-fed beef. Recent studies also show that CLA (conjugated linoleic acid) and TVA (trans-vaccenic acid) are present in grass-fed beef but may not be found in the grocer's version. These two acids have been flying off the health food store shelves for the last ten years as supplements to fight cancer and cardiovascular disease—two illnesses that have plagued our nation since the industrial era.

Raising cows is to your benefit no matter how you look at it, which breed you choose, or what your preferred purpose might be. You'll find a rich and rewarding experience plus far healthier food for everyone in your family.

Choosing a Breed to Raise

Cattle come in a wide variety of breeds and crossbreeds classified as purebred dairy breeds (registered or non-registered), meat breeds, crossbreeds, dual-purpose breeds, or miniatures.

Dairy and beef breeds are just that. They may have been developed over a few years or a few centuries and they have one specific purpose—either to produce milk at top quantities or to grow quickly with a high meat-to-bone ratio.

Crossbreeds are used most often as beef cattle. These cattle have been bred purposefully—either to thrive in their environment or as an attempt to create a new and better meat breed. Dependent on your objective a crossbreed might be the best animal for your money. Especially so if you aren't interested in establishing a show-quality or registered herd.

Finally, and worthy of consideration, are the smaller dual-purpose cattle and miniatures. In every other section of this book I've avoided the novelty, the toy, and the fancy breeds, but in cattle the dual-purpose and miniature cattle cannot be ignored based on their service to the small family farmer.

Dairy Breeds

Before you run off to buy a family milker, consider this: the average dairy cow provides twenty to twenty-four quarts of milk every day, three hundred or more days of the year. Consistent yields are realized by keeping one of the top six milk breeds.

Standard dairy cows mature between 900 and 1,500 pounds; bulls and steers, between 1,500 and 2,000 pounds. The most popular dairy breeds are, listed from smallest to largest, Jersey, Guernsey, Ayrshire, Milking Shorthorn, Brown Swiss, and Holstein.

Your decision on which breed to raise might be made based on local availability, quality of pasture, and climate conditions. While all milk breeds are hardy enough to thrive in most North American climates, some may do better than others in your area. Discussions with local ranchers, veterinarians, or your feed supply store are highly beneficial.

The two smallest dairy breeds, the Jersey and the Guernsey, each have an interesting trait that you should know about before selecting them as your breed of choice. Jersey calves sold for beef will net low prices should you plan to sell them. Even though the beef is as tasty as any other, the fat of the meat is yellow, which the marketplace misjudges as "less than fresh." Even a Jersey cross shows yellow-colored fat. The Guernsey, on the other hand, has milk that is a slightly yellow to cream color. This shouldn't present a problem unless you have some real finicky eaters at your dining table.

Beef Breeds

Although any breed of cattle can be raised for beef, some breeds are widely recognized for their good mothering instincts, fast growth, having small calves (small calves equates to easier births), and climatic hardiness.

Hundreds of beef breeds and crossbreeds exist in North America and any purebred or crossbred calf will yield delicious, nutritious, and economical beef under your control within just a few months. If your plan is just to raise one or two calves for the freezer, check the sales of breeds readily available in your area and choose the healthiest calf you can find from the most knowledge-able or recommended seller.

Generally speaking, beef and crossbred calves are forty-five to fifty pounds at birth and kept on pasture with their mothers for the summer and most of the fall. They will have cost little to raise but will provide 320 to 380 pounds of beef for the freezer given that they have reached their seven-month potential of 600 to 650 pounds live weight.

Dual-Purpose and Miniature Breeds

Although there are many dual-purpose breeds in North America, the most popular is the Dexter breed. These smallish cattle reach maturity at 750 and 900 pounds, standing thirty-six and forty-two inches tall at the shoulder, for cows and bulls respectively.

A good Dexter cow will supply one to three gallons of milk per day (a manageable amount compared to her Holstein counterpart of five to six gallons daily). Her offspring at seven to eight months of age will grow to be 350 to 500 pounds, 55 to 60 percent of which will end up in your freezer.

Although the Dexter is a small breed, it isn't considered a mini-ature by all breeders. In fact, the rules and boundaries between dual-purpose and miniatures are somewhat fuzzy across developers and registries.

Miniature cattle are not the latest fad. Documentation of smaller cattle has been noted since the late 1960s, and at present time there are nearly thirty registered breeds—ranging from the original Dexters and Zebu (from Ireland and Mexico respectively) to the American-made Lowline (a miniature version of the Angus).

These cattle are a viable, useful, and productive alternative for the small families who keep them. It is no longer necessary to be overwhelmed by the massive output of a full-sized breed or to be stuck trying to find friends to share the bounty of milk and split a side of beef with you.

Temperament and Training of Cattle

Dairy cows and beef cattle are herd animals. They settle into a new home most easily when they are with their own kind and have less tendency to be nervous. A lone calf will bond with you and consider you one of the herd if you are quick to understand its needs and its nature.

Calves and mature cattle can be timid if they've been raised on pasture and are not accustomed to human interaction. Even if they were, you as the new owner will not be "their" human until they have spent ample time with you. As long as they have been treated fairly in the past and you give them a little grace and space in the beginning, you'll have them ambling over to greet you in the field or pen in no time.

All cattle have vivid, long-lasting memories that serve them to associate both painful and pleasurable situations with a person, place, or inanimate object. You can tap into that ability once you understand it. You can train youngsters to respect the electric fence or give you space, for instance, as well as teaching them a call word that will have them running back home for grain at top speeds.

The best manner to tame and raise cattle is with a gentle and steady temperament. Cow and steer alike can neither tolerate nor learn to trust the human who is flailing his arms, screeching and yelling, or rushing at them. You should not be so mild-mannered that you let them walk all over you either. Once you've gained their trust, the next step is to assert and establish yourself as a respect-worthy herd "boss."

Every calf, heifer, steer, and cow also has his or her own self-defined comfort zone. By respecting you, they will understand and learn your own comfort zone and therefore will be less likely to crowd or push you, step on your feet, or trample you in a moment of panic. To teach them about your boundaries you'll have to give them a sharp rap on the nose or the hindquarters with a small stick. This not only gets their attention but also lets them know that they have come too close or that their behavior is unacceptable.

If an intentional, well-placed smack doesn't stop them in their tracks, you haven't hit hard enough. These are heavily muscled animals with thick hides. At 1,000 pounds, they can certainly push you over or crush your entire foot if they are not taught to

BELOW: Stay calm and prepare to be the herd boss to ensure that your cow respects your space.

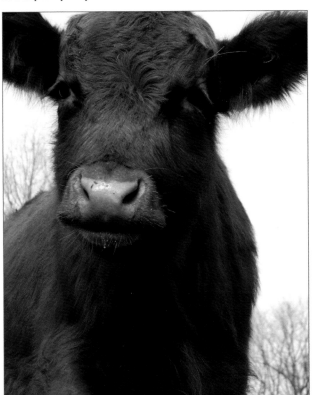

respect your space. I never condone abuse of an animal, but cattle can easily put you in the hospital, in a cast, or in a wheelchair. One sharp smack does not constitute abuse.

One final point about the temperament of cattle: their shyness can induce panic, and there is nothing safe about a half-ton animal in a panic. Calves panic if they cannot find their mothers and will run circles, risk their own lives, and cry for hours in frustration. Mature cattle will panic if cornered. In that situation and without being controlled they will mow down anything or anyone to get themselves out of the fearful situation.

Train a calf to lead by a halter and you can keep that panic at bay at any age. They will have learned that once in the halter their panic serves no purpose—the human on the other side of the rope is in control. Even with an animal of this size under control, you should never let your guard down. Keep a plan of escape and stay out of the kick zone whenever you're working with one, on or off the halter.

Designing Your Small Farm Strategy

Milk and Meat Yields for Cows

Although widely ranging in size, approximate yields to be expected from raising cattle are as follows:

- Dairy—Average milk supply of 1,500 to 1,800 gallons per year.
- Beef—60 percent of live weight can be expected as dressed and packaged beef.
- Dairy Breeds Raised for Beef—A dairy heifer calf, raised just seven months, weighs between 350 and 450 pounds (netting 190 to 260 pounds of beef). If you raise her another year to 700 to 1,000 pounds, your freezer beef doubles. Add 30 percent if raising a dairy steer for beef.

- Beef Breeds Raised for Beef—A heifer calf at weaning will
  weigh between 450 and 600 pounds (netting 270 to 360
  pounds of beef). Raised to maturity, the heifer weighs
  900 to 1,000 pounds. Again, add 30 percent when raising
  steers.

A few options in raising cattle for a food source are listed below. Choose or alter one of the strategies below to suit your needs, space, and time. Keep in mind that the family milk cow is the animal that, once owned, must be tended to on a schedule. Twice daily milking, twelve hours apart, seven days a week. To put her off is to decrease her value and in some cases jeopardize her health.

- Keep and breed a dairy cow every year for up to six gallons of
  milk per day, plus one calf to either sell or raise until late fall
  for approximately 250 pounds of dressed beef in the freezer.
- Keep and breed a dairy cow every year and once she has
  calved, purchase up to three orphaned calves for her to
  raise with her own. Your cow will produce enough milk to
  nurse four calves. Once they are weaned, they can be sold
  or put to pasture until late fall and you'll still have an ample
  milk supply for your family for another seven months.
  These four calves plus six months on pasture could yield
  1,000 pounds of beef.
- Keep and breed a dairy cow every year with a beef breed
  bull. The resulting calf will be smaller at birth but quick
  to grow on pasture. His crossbred capability could net you
  350 pounds or more of beef for the freezer, plus all the milk
  your family can drink for seven months or more.
- Keep one or more beef cattle on pasture and butcher when
  the season ends for a quick freezer full of beef (an average of
  four hundred pounds of dressed beef). Alternatively, winter
  the animal and raise him on to next fall to double your yield
  for less than the cost of a hundred square bales of hay.
- Raise dual-purpose or miniature cattle for realistic and
  manageable output of milk and/or beef, especially if available
  pasture is minimal.

Pens, Pasture, and Shelter

Newborn calves should be kept in a warm and clean barn or shed for at least three weeks. This small calf has the potential for many stress-related sicknesses severe enough to take her life. Ensure that the calf cannot escape, cannot damage herself within her surroundings, has clean bedding in a draft-free enclosure, is treated gently and compassionately, and is receiving adequate nutrition.

The started or newly weaned calf would also have the best start on your farm when kept in a barn for a week or more with similar conditions. Although young dairy calves are at greater risk than beef, both will attempt to escape back to their dams.

Outdoor Pens

Should you choose to move or start an older calf in an outdoor pen, the fencing around the pen will need to be both tight and tall,

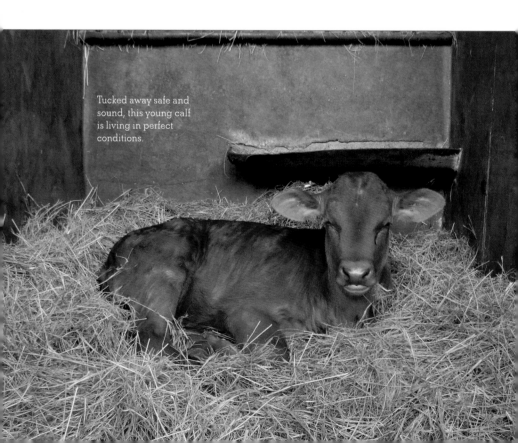

Tucked away safe and sound, this young calf is living in perfect conditions.

especially if you are only raising one calf. You'll also need to provide a shelter from cold winds and scorching suns, but the shelter can be moved onto pasture with the calf when you decide to do so.

The standard confinement pen built to take a weaned calf to seven months of age should be at least 1,000 square feet in size. The perimeter should be constructed of thinly spaced, well-supported wire or wood planks. If you plan eventually to pasture the calf, wait until she has settled into her new farm and owners before training her on the electric fence.

Additional Calves

Plan on raising more than one calf in an outdoor pen? You don't need to double the space for every calf you add. One thousand square feet for the first calf plus 250 square feet for every additional calf is all that is required. Be sure to increase bedding and shade area for every calf added as well.

Inside the pen include a three-sided and roofed shed in one corner for bedding, a hay manger, and a salt/mineral block. The shed should be at least one hundred square feet in size and cleaned daily. The water bucket or tub can be set into an adjacent corner and blocked in at eighteen to twenty inches off the ground to ensure the calf doesn't spill, step in, or soil the water.

The Pasture

The pasture requirement for growing cattle is one and a half to two and a half acres each. Miniatures only require one half acre each. In winter months or slow growing seasons you'll need to supplement pasture with hay, and in some situations, a bit of grain.

All cattle require a shaded area. This could be a large stand of trees, but it is better if they have access to a roofed, three-sided shelter. The shaded area needs to be dry at all times and checked regularly for waste removal. Cows, steers, and calves should never be expected to stand or lie down in wet or filthy conditions.

If you have adequate acreage, employ rotational pasturing. Controlling which area of the land your cow pastures will ensure that new growth is eaten evenly.

Pasture fencing will need to be reinforced by electric wire. Cows are quite capable of mowing over any flimsy barrier in a panic. Even a herd that has been taught to respect a powerful electric fence will have heifers in heat eager to crash through in search of a mate. Woven wire cattle fence, forty-seven inches high with a strand above and below of electric fencing, has worked well on our farm.

Finding a Calf or Cow to Purchase

Some years are better than others for purchasing calves or a milking cow. The same can be said for seasons. You are most likely to find dairy calves for sale in the spring and beef breed calves selling in the fall. Before you make any purchase, read up a little on the breed (or breeds if you're considering a crossbred) available for sale. Take some time to observe other herds in the field, in pictures on the Internet, or at country fairs and auctions. When the time comes to make your purchase, drag along a knowledgeable friend or ask a veterinarian for advice.

Disposition, if it can be sized up in a mere ten minutes of observation, should also be considered. Healthy calves are alert, energetic, and have bright shining eyes. High-strung calves are always to be avoided as are the dim-witted ones. If you have a few to choose from, select an alert and mellow calf. He will gain more weight and be easier to handle than his larger, wild, and snorty herdmate. Steer clear of calves showing any signs of illness such as runny stools, dripping noses, and crusty eyes.

Dairy Calves

Commercial dairies breed to freshen their cows for another year of milk production. As a result, every spring the dairies are faced with a glut of calves to dispose of. Some smaller dairies breed their calves with a meat bull known to throw small calves. This is beneficial. You could wind up with a crossbred, meatier calf to raise.

The hardship of raising excess dairy stock is that they'll only be a few hours or days old when you purchase them. These calves will require bottle-feeding, scrupulous living conditions, and a watchful eye for any sign of stress or illness. Dairy bull calves sell the cheapest. The heifers, if turned out well, might make a nice dual-purpose crossbred that you decide to keep for the long term as a low-quantity milk source.

Should you decide to purchase spring calves, do so directly from the dairy and not from a livestock auction. Spring calves are more susceptible to picking up viruses—not to mention the stress of moving twice in one day. A direct-from-dairy purchase is a faster transport for a stressed calf and you can purchase enough colostrum for your calf's first week. After the first week these young calves are fed milk replacer, purchased from your local feed store.

Beef Calves

The second norm for calf sales is in the fall when beef cattle ranchers sell freshly weaned calves off the field. These calves will be well established and less susceptible to disease, will have naturally picked up antibodies from their mothers' milk, and are already castrated and disbudded. Weaned calves should also have all orders of business taken care of including first vaccinations.

Although physically established, they may be a little more difficult to handle until they gain your trust. They are much larger than newborn dairy calves and will take a little extra time to train. There will be stress with the move to their new home, but it will not be as devastating or potentially life-threatening for this calf.

Mature Dairy Cows

On occasion throughout the year, you may luck upon an established and bred milking cow for sale. This may be a single sale or the result of a small dairy changing their business model. Local newspapers, the feed store, classified ad sites on the Internet, and your own network of friends are some of the avenues to explore. Good dairy cows are in their top production between four and nine years of age, and will continue to serve you for another three to eight years after.

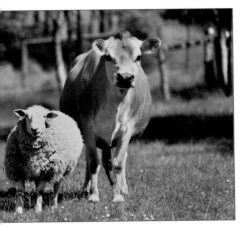

ABOVE: Cows and sheep will keep each other company when they don't have one of their own kind nearby.

Mature cows are more expensive but might be a great bargain from an honest seller. You'll have access to barn records (or at the very least be able to ask questions about milking and calving history) and the option to "try before you buy." Not all milking cows are suitable and comfortable for all hands and skill level, after all.

Finally, don't be shy. There isn't one farmer I know of that takes offense to a stranger knocking on his or her door or leaving a note in the mailbox saying, "I'd like to buy one of your heifers or steers." Even if he doesn't have one for sale, he probably knows another farmer who is eager to lighten his herd by one or two.

Feed Requirements

Cattle do well on good pasture with a mineral salt block. Seldom is anything more required. Calves, dairy cows, and cattle en route to market are the exceptions.

Hay that is suitable for cows and cattle is a combination of legume (alfalfa and clover) and grass hay. If the legume quantity in hay is inadequate you can add a little cottonseed, soybean, or linseed meal to their diets until you find a better hay provider. Talk to your local feed supply store or veterinarian for recommendations or advice if you're unsure about the quality of your pasture or hay.

A salt block intended for cattle or a mineral salt block combination ensures your cattle are getting the required amounts of trace elements and vitamins. If your region or pasture is known to be deficient in iodine and selenium it may be added in the local salt blocks you purchase.

Grain and sweet feed (grain mixed with molasses) are used only for weight gain or to supplement a very poor-quality hay. Corn, milo, oats, wheat, and barley are all acceptable grains for cows when used in moderation.

A producing dairy cow is given one half to one pound of 16 percent protein grain for every quart of milk that she produces, after the first week of calving. The quantity of grain required to keep her producing to her maximum will change throughout the year. Keep barn records to monitor and adjust grain ration accordingly.

Hay fed to dairy calves should be fine-stemmed and leafy. Almost any other good quality hay is fine for the rest of the herd. By the time a dairy calf is three months old she should be eating two to four pounds of growing ration containing 15 to 18 percent protein and three pounds of hay per day for every one hundred pounds she weighs.

Beef calves are usually on the field and following their mother's example of grazing. Until they are weaned they are not likely to have ever eaten grain. Grain is usually reserved for beef steers and heifers to help them achieve their top weight before going to market. Changes to their feed should be gradual and never should they be fed a diet consisting only of grain.

Water

All cattle should have access to fresh, clean water at all times. There is never an exception to this rule. One beef breed steer or heifer will drink twenty-five to fifty gallons of water a day; a dairy cow, from fifteen to twenty gallons. This changes with the seasons, the freshness of pasture, and whether or not the cow is in production.

Winter Feeding and Bedding

You'll save money and the last-minute scurry of trying to find hay for sale if you buy freshly baled hay off the field. You can pick it up yourself, one pickup load at a time, or pay someone to collect and deliver it to your farm.

Check hay before storing to ensure it has dried and is not wet or moldy. Moldy hay is of no use to livestock. Hay should be stored off the ground and protected from sun, rain, and snow. Stack it as

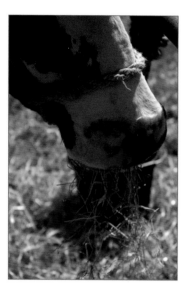

high as you can on skids and only uncover what you'll need for each day. If the hay is dusty from the field, give it a good fluff and shake before feeding to your cattle.

A mature cow will eat twenty-five to thirty pounds of hay per day during the winter months. The average square bale of hay weighs forty-five pounds. Therefore one dairy cow from November 1 to March 1 will consume 3,600 pounds of hay, or 80 bales (120 days times 30 pounds divided by 45-pound bales). These are assumptive and general guidelines; adjust your winter hay needs to suit your cow and climate.

While you're at the chore of purchasing hay for the winter, you might also prepare for bedding material before the weather turns cold. One cow's bedding matter often accounts for another five pounds of matter per day whether in the form of straw or wood shavings.

Cattle Health

Buying healthy animals, keeping their bedding clean, feeding quality hay, providing clean water, and adhering to a veterinary-approved vaccination schedule will go a long way in keeping your cattle healthy.

Keeping herd, dairy, or barn notes can also be beneficial should any of your animals fall ill. Quick access to vaccination records, changes in feed, and first signs of behavioral changes all help to assess and treat any illness or disease. Also, should you one day plan to sell your cow, calf, or cattle, you'll have records of progress, production, and maintenance readily accessible for the new buyer. (A sample health record for cattle can be found in the forms section at the end of this book.)

Vaccinations

All cattle should be vaccinated by a veterinarian to address nation-wide and region-specific diseases. This is not just to protect the animal, but to protect your investment and your own health if you are raising livestock to provide food for the table.

Common vaccinations include infectious bovine rhinotra-cheitis, bovine virus diarrhea, parainfluenza, blackleg, malignant edema, brucellosis, and leptospirosis. Vaccination schedules may start as early as a few months of age.

Signs of Trouble

If you have spent any time with your cattle you will be the first to notice subtle changes in their health and behavior. Lying down for longer periods, being off feed, kicking at his own belly, lack of interest in surroundings, and restlessness are all subtle signs that the animal is not feeling well.

Cow, Steer, and Calf Vital Signs

- Rectal temperature: 101.5 degrees Fahrenheit
- Pulse rate: Forty to seventy beats per minute
- Breathing rate: Beef, ten to thirty breaths per minute; dairy, eighteen to twenty-eight
- Heifer puberty: Ten to twelve months of age, dependent on breed
- Average birth weight: Thirty-five to forty-five pounds
- Average gestation period: 276 to 294 days
- Heat cycle: Every nineteen to twenty-three days
- Heat period: Twelve to eighteen hours

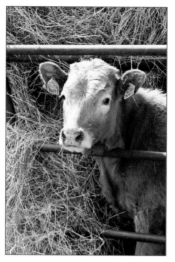

Keeping Barn Records

It makes good sense to keep a record of important facts about every calf or cattle on your farm. This assists you during sale of any animal as well as keeping track of health issues, vaccinations, expected calving dates, and milk production. A sample form with an ample margin for notes is available at the back of this book to photocopy and use. Alternatively, download blank 9 x 11-inch forms from www.KeepingFarmAnimals.com

Common Diseases and Illnesses

Some of the most common illnesses that affect cattle are listed below. While some are preventable through vaccination, others listed here are just part and parcel of raising cattle. If no cure is listed below, then none has been found to date. Always consult with a veterinarian before treating, self-diagnosing, or culling an animal.

Common Illnesses

Abscess

Also known as lumpy jaw as this oral bacterial infection results in large abscesses on the side of the face or jaw.

Treatment: A veterinarian must puncture and drain the abscess and may prescribe antibiotics.

Acidosis

Brought on by too much grain resulting in overproduction of lactic acid. A calf may show fever, diarrhea, and founder (see below).

Prevention: A managed feed schedule and accessibility to clean water at all times.

Treatment: Call the veterinarian if you think your calf has acidosis for immediate treatment.

Blackleg
A bacterial disease that causes a sudden sickness leading to death.
Prevention: Vaccination at two months of age and a follow-up vaccination at weaning. The vaccine is preventative against other clostridial diseases (brought on by organisms in the soil) including red water, tetanus, malignant edema, and entero-toxemia. Your veterinarian will have the correct and updated clostridial vaccination for your region.

Bloat
A digestive problem most often brought on by feed fermentation in the gut. Frothy gas builds up in the stomach and puts so much pressure on the animal's lungs it cannot breathe. Swelling can be seen on the left side of an animal with bloat.
Prevention: Potentially fermenting feeds such as alfalfa pasture, alfalfa hay, and grain should be given in moderation.
Treatment: Immediate veterinarian assistance will be required to save the animal's life.

Brucellosis
Also known as Bang's disease. Only heifers and cows are affected. Infection causes the abortion of calves, most often between five to eight months of pregnancy. Milk from a carrier or infected cow causes undulant fever in humans.
Prevention: Vaccination between two and ten months of age. Vaccinated heifers receive a tag and a tattoo as proof of vaccination.

Cancer Eye
Starts as a small sore on the eye or surrounding skin. Most often seen in white-faced cattle lacking pigment in the skin around the eyes.

Treatment: The only treatment is surgical removal by a qualified veterinarian.

Coccidiosis

An intestinal disease picked up through contaminated water or dirty living conditions.

Treatment: Progressive symptoms of severe and bloody diarrhea can only be treated by a veterinarian. Some animals may be carriers and never show signs of the disease.

Diarrhea (Scours)

Calf scours can be viral, bacterial, or parasitic and can affect calves from two days up to a year of age. Newborn calves suffer the worst and often cannot be treated quickly enough to be saved.

Treatment: Call the veterinarian. The cause must first be discovered before the calf can be treated. Electrolyte fluids and antibiotics are often prescribed as well as forced feeding through an esophageal feeder. It is best if the calf can nurse regularly, but if it will not, the esophageal feeder must be used. Chances of cure without a veterinarian's assistance are minimal.

Diphtheria

A throat infection brought on by the same organisms that cause foot rot (below), diphtheria causes difficulty in breathing and eating, a fever, cough, and drool. The swelling inside the mouth will obstruct air and feed intake if not treated quickly.

Treatment: Veterinarian-prescribed antibiotics.

Foot Rot

Foot rot is a bacterial infection brought on through entry of a wound in the foot.

Prevention: Keep calves and cattle off of wet, muddy land.

Treatment: Veterinarian-prescribed antibiotics.

Founder

A painful and serious affliction that causes the hoof wall to separate from the foot causing malformation and lameness.

Treatment: Immediate veterinary attention is required.

Hardware Disease

Also known as traumatic reticulopericarditis. The consumption of metal objects including sharp wires and nails that eventually puncture the reticulum and vital organs.

Prevention: Keep stalls and pastures free of debris. Some farmers feed their cattle small magnets to bind any metal objects to the reticulum before causing any further distress.

Treatment: In case of infection caused by a reticulum puncture, antibiotics may be effective.

Leptospirosis

A bacterial disease spread by contaminated feed or water. The disease is usually spread by mice or other wildlife and even by infected domestic livestock and pets.

Prevention: Part of annual or biannual vaccinations for heifers and cows.

Lymphoma

Also known as lymphosarcoma. A viral infection caused by BLV (bovine leukemia virus). Although hard to spot by the untrained eye, enlarged lymph nodes, infertility, loss of health, and bulging eyes are common signals.

Mastitis

A painful bacterial infection in the udder. The udder will feel hot and milk may have signs of lumps or streaks of blood.

Prevention: Keep all milking equipment, including your hands, clean. Apply a teat dip after every milking session. Once a month check your cow with a mastitis test.

Treatment: Antibiotics might be in order. Milk your cow every two to three hours if the case is mild, watching carefully that the infection doesn't worsen. Your cow's immune system may clear up the infection. Dispose of any milk. If antibiotics are used, consult with your veterinarian for a clear date.

Paratuberculosis

Also known as Johne's disease. A bacterial infection that causes chronic diarrhea and a slow and methodical wasting of the animal.

Prevention: No vaccine exists and no treatment of the animal is possible. The only option is to cull the animal and have every other animal on your property tested.

Pinkeye

A contagious bacterial infection caused by face flies. The affected animal develops watery eyes and will hold the affected eye shut. A growing white spot will be seen on the cornea of the infected eye.

Treatment: An antibiotic powder or spray that must be administered at least twice per day. Although pinkeye may clear up on its own, it is recommended to treat the condition promptly.

Pneumonia

Although cattle of any age can contract pneumonia, it is the number two killer of young calves. Various bacteria and viruses attack a calf that is either stressed or has a low immune system. Signs of illness are runny nose, coughing, lack of interest in feed and surroundings, lying down or standing hunched, and fast respiration.

Prevention: Lessen stress factors of a newborn or young calf by any means necessary. Older cattle should not be overcrowded, subjected to long periods of wet and coldness, poor ventilation, or less than clean living conditions.

Treatment: Call your veterinarian for immediate antibiotic treatment if fever is over 102.5 degrees Fahrenheit.

Ringworm

A fungal infection most often spread to the entire herd. Passed on through repeated rubbing against the same post and recognized by one- to two-inch circles of missing hair with patchy dry skin underneath.

Prevention: Contagious to humans. Wash thoroughly after contact with infected animals.

Treatment: Veterinarian assistance may be utilized, but it generally clears up on its own by spring. Discuss milk safety with your veterinarian if treating dairy cattle, as a topical fungicide may be effective.

Selenium Deficiency

Also known as white muscle disease and nutritional myopathy. Affected calves may be too weak to move after birth or die from heart failure after exercise, and heifers may abort during pregnancy.

Prevention: Know if there is a selenium deficiency in your region. Heifers and cows should receive a selenium shot in their seventh month of pregnancy, as well as newborn calves in extreme cases.

Internal and External Parasites

Lice and flies can cause a decrease in the health of your cow or cattle. Lice are most common in the cooler winter months and make an animal itchy to the point of hair loss. To rid your herd of lice you'll need a powder or liquid safe for dairy or beef cattle and available from the feed store or veterinarian. Follow the directions on the package and be sure to reapply in time to catch lice eggs unaffected by the treatment that hatch over the next ten days.

Heel flies can also cause serious troubles in your cattle as they lay eggs on the lower portion

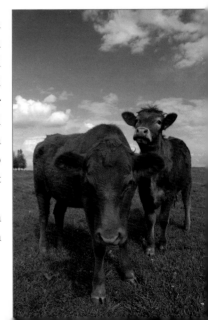

of your cow's legs, and when the grub hatches it travels through the body, under the skin of the animal. An insecticidal product for heel flies (also known as cattle grubs or warbles) is also available from the veterinarian or feed supply store.

Horn flies and face flies bite cattle, infect their eyes with pinkeye, and are an annoyance. Insecticidal ear tags are now available for cattle, which lessens the problem considerably.

As with any animal on pasture, cattle are susceptible to intestinal worms and parasites. You can tell if an animal is infested by its dull, rough coat, poor appetite, and diarrhea, or through a stool sample tested by your veterinarian. Medication will be required.

Breeding for Milk Flow or Beef Calves

Many heifers will reach puberty by their first birthday, but shouldn't be bred until they are fifteen months old. This ensures they don't calve until they are two years old. If breeding a beef heifer, her weight is as important as her age. She should reach 65 percent of the expected mature weight for her breed.

Before breeding, ensure vaccinations are up to date—many of the antibodies in her system will be passed to her calf in the uterus and through first milk consumption. Talk to your veterinarian as soon as you know your animal has been bred to discuss her vaccination schedule, including the newer anti-scour vaccinations.

As long as you aren't planning on raising or selling purebred, registered calves you can breed your heifer or cow with any available bull. The best bull is one that is historically known for throwing small birth-weight calves—especially so if this will be her first calf. The second-best bull is one that lives in the field next door and whose owner doesn't mind a free rendezvous between the two. Taking the time to find an appropriate bull for first breeding is a worthy pursuit. A calf that grows too large in an immature uterus may die at birth or cause physical damage to your heifer.

Signs of Heat

Most heifers and mature cows have no trouble letting you know they are in heat. They will pace at the fence line, bawl to ensure any bull within five miles knows she is ready to breed, and, if other cattle are in the field, either attempt to mount them or allow them to mount her. If your heifer or cow does not display these outward signs, check her regularly for mucus on her back end—a sure sign she is in heat. A heat will only last twelve to eighteen hours. The most opportune time to breed her is in the later half of those hours. Non-bred heifers and cows will return to heat every twenty-one days.

The Pregnancy

Cattle carry their young for nine months (285 days, give or take 9 days on either side). Watch your heifer closely during a first pregnancy for correct weight gain and nutrition. Not only will she be supplying nutrition to the growing fetus, but she'll also still be growing herself. This first pregnancy could affect the remainder of her life and every future pregnancy. Ensuring that she is in top physical health almost guarantees a safe delivery, ample milk for the newborn, and successful breeding in later years.

Nutrition of the Bred Heifer

When pasture growth slows, add a nutrient-rich protein source to her diet. Alfalfa hay is the easiest, most affordable way to add protein, calcium, and Vitamin A to her diet. Throughout the duration of the pregnancy, continue to feed both alfalfa and grass hay.

You only need to supplement her feed with grain if she is losing weight or if the hay you're feeding her is insufficient. Grain will not make up for a shortcoming in nutrients, nor will it keep her warm during cold spells. The digestion of extra hay, not grain, adds warmth to cattle. Your feed store may carry a nutrition-packed feed designed with bred heifers in mind, which may be better than straight grain from the bag.

Awaiting Delivery

Cows that have already calved should be dried off two months before a new calf is due. Heifers might benefit from some practice time on the stanchions. Feed her a little grain, restrain and brush her, then wash her udder and teats. By the time she calves the milking routine will be old hat to her.

While her due date approaches, prepare a place for her to safely calve and gather the supplies you might need on delivery. If this will be your first calving experience, your veterinarian's emergency phone number is a must, as well as a few experienced and local friends' numbers.

Calves can be born on the field or in a barn stall as long as the area is clean and dry. Pasture births should only be allowed if the weather is warm and the cow can be safely alone in a grass-covered, shady spot. Stall births require ample room for the cow to move around comfortably, a non-slippery floor, and clean bedding.

Supplies you might need include:

- Strong iodine solution for the calf's navel
- Clean towels to dry the calf off
- A baby bottle with a lamb nipple in case you need to feed the calf
- Long, disposable gloves in case you need to right the calf in the birth canal
- Fitted halter and rope to restrain or lead your cow or heifer
- Half-inch nylon rope in case you need to pull the calf out of the birth canal

All heifers and cows are different, but any time between a few weeks and a few hours before labor, she may show a full udder with dripping teats, an enlarged vulva, an active tail, and restless behavior. As the moment draws near you may see signs of contractions and her noticeable desire for seclusion. When birth is imminent (twenty minutes to two hours away), a flush of yellow water, the

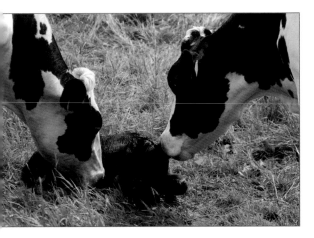

LEFT: As cows are inquisitive, not much time passes after a new birth before other cows in the herd pay their respects and meet the new addition.

unbroken water sac, or tiny hooves will appear. Most deliveries are trouble-free without human intervention, but if an hour has passed without progress, call the veterinarian for help.

Heifers and cows often lie down for the remainder of the delivery. You can leave her where she lies as long as the calf won't be obstructed during delivery. Once the calf has fully arrived it should either be breathing or your cow should be attentive to the lack of breath. Give her ample time to attend to the task herself, but by all means step in if she doesn't seem to notice the calf. Remove the sac from the calf's face and tickle his nostril to get a sneeze out of him. The sneeze alone should alert your cow enough to take over the remainder of care, but if not, the next step in newborn care is to dry him off completely and gently rub him all over to get his circulation pumping.

If you have time between all this and the moment the calf stands to nurse, wash your cow's udder and teats with warm water only. A calf should be nursing by thirty minutes or, as might be the case with a difficult birth, up to two hours later. You can step in and help cow and calf by standing him up, nose to a teat, and supporting him until he has drunk as much as he will take. If he doesn't appear interested or your cow is being difficult, milk her and feed him by baby bottle.

At some point during the next hour you'll need to treat the umbilical cord and navel stump. The optimum length for a navel stump is three inches, but longer is fine as long as it isn't dragging on the ground. Do not touch the stump, as germs and bacteria are easily passed into the calf's system this way. Dip the stump completely into a small cup filled with iodine. Bull calves will need to have an iodine dip repeated numerous times throughout the first day as they will sully the stump every time they urinate.

Your cow may take a few hours to shed the afterbirth. Once expelled, remove and dispose of it. If it has not expelled completely or at all, do not intervene without veterinary assistance.

First Milk

The first five to six milking sessions after delivery are colostrum, a rich and heavy milk loaded with fats and antibodies intended to increase disease resistance and assist calves with their first bowel movements. One to two good feeds of colostrum will provide all a newborn calf needs to get started on the right foot. By the seventh to eighth day, colostrum is completely replaced by milk suitable for human consumption.

Storing Colostrum

Colostrum can be milked and frozen for many years with minimal loss of nutrients and benefits. Store a gallon or two, clearly marked, and you'll have some on hand to start orphan calves in later years.

If you're raising a dairy cow, the first nurse is your chance to make some dairy management decisions.

Dairy cows generate enough milk to support up to four calves—or at the very least enough for your entire family plus the calf. Consider these options:

- Remove the calf from the cow, milk the cow to feed to the calf by bottle, and commit to bottle-feeding for the next three months.
- Separate cow and calf after first feeding, then allow the calf to nurse from the front teats twice per day while you simultaneously collect milk in a bucket off the rear teats.
- Quickly purchase newborn orphaned calves (from a dairy farm eager to sell freshening calves) and raise them all on your cow's milk by bottle or train the cow to accept each one as her own.

Should you decide to take a more natural route—allowing calf to stay with cow—consider that one of the primary reasons a farmer separates the two is to protect the cow's udder. A cow's udder may be swollen or caked inside after calving. Repeated bunting from a boisterous calf during the first few days of milk flow can cause irreparable damage. Manual milking protects the cow's sensitive udder until her milk flows easily.

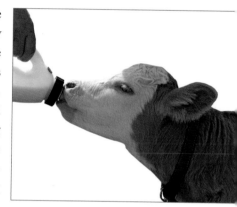

If or when you return the calf to cow, begin milking her twice daily, twelve hours apart, to ease udder pressure (one calf will not be able to drink all the milk she's producing) and ensure that every quarter has been emptied.

Dairy Calf Milestones and Management

By one week of age you can add a small piece of starter ration into your calf's mouth after each feeding to help him acquire a taste for it. At three weeks of age he can nibble on fine-leafed hay but he won't eat much of it until he is about eight weeks of age. Sometime between the eighth and twelfth week he can be fully weaned from teat or bottle.

As long as the calf is doing nicely by three weeks of age you can attend to horn buds, scrotal sacs, and extra teats.

Bull calves, once castrated, become steers that are easier to manage and provide tastier beef. Castration is a simple task, causing only minimal discomfort to the calf as long as it is attended to early in life. Using an Elastrator, a tightening ring is attached over the scrotum, which causes the testicles inside to die. No bleeding, just a small tender area that disappears within a month's time. Staff at the feed store—or wherever you purchase your Elastrator—can instruct you on precise use, but instructions also come with the device.

Unless the calf you are raising is a horned-breed purebred, it is best to remove horns when the calf is young. Up to three months of age an electric disbudding iron may be used and takes just a few minutes per calf to perform. Caustic paste can be used on newborn calves (up to three days) but this method isn't without tragedies and is far less popular than the electric disbudding irons of today.

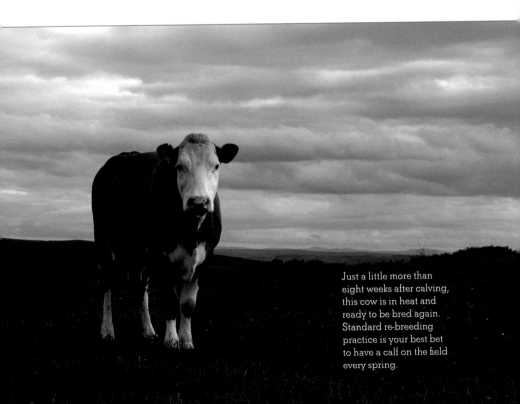

Just a little more than eight weeks after calving, this cow is in heat and ready to be bred again. Standard re-breeding practice is your best bet to have a calf on the field every spring.

Some heifer calves are born with five or six teats instead of four. The extras serve no use and might even cause her trouble as she ages. Between two and four weeks of age you should be able to easily tell which are the main teats and which are extras. Extra teats are most often found close to one of the main four teats. To remove one, disinfect your hands, scissors, and the teat, then snip from front to back (lengthwise with the body frame) at the point where teat meets udder. Nothing more than a swab of iodine is required after removal. (Do not perform this task if you are unsure or if the heifer calf is any older than four weeks. Call a veterinarian.)

Vaccinations

Within your calf's first month, schedule an appointment with your veterinarian for first vaccinations. Some are given as early as two months of age and may include selenium injections to ensure your calf's nutritional needs are met.

To Breed Again

Your cow will soon come into heat again. You'll know when she's ready to be bred by her usual signs. She may also give a lot less milk on the day she's in heat. Cows are rebred on their first or second heat sixty days past calving. This breeding practice ensures she has a full year between calves and the milk keeps flowing for most of the year.

How to Milk a Cow

A dairy cow, like a milk goat, thrives on routine. They need to see you at the same times every day, preferably twelve hours apart.

The major difference between the cow and doe however, is that a cow can refuse you—even when her milk is overflowing and the udder pressure unbearable. She may have a reason to refuse to let down her milk, but you can work around her reasoning even if she doesn't cooperate. The solution is in finding the trigger that counteracts her stubbornness—a natural hormone, oxytocin.

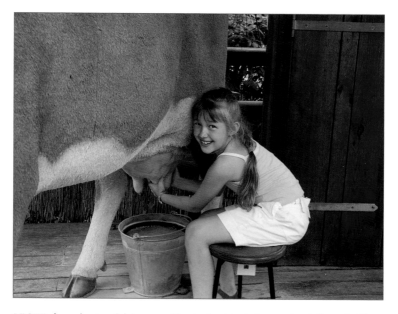

ABOVE: A good-natured dairy cow will arrive back to the barn, twice daily, and will stand without stanchions while anyone milks her.

Milk flow will commence within a minute of an oxytocin release, often stimulated by any act that she associates with giving milk. Triggers might be a feed of grain at the stanchions, being brushed, seeing a milking stool or pail, or an udder wash. In fact the very act of washing her udder and teats with warm water will bring on a flow of milk that even the smartest cow cannot stop. The trouble with this flow is that you only have eight to ten minutes before she's back in control of her own body again.

Cleanliness of your cow and all equipment (including hers) should be your top concern. Sanitize all equipment before and after milking, including udder and teats.

The practice and treatment of obtaining and storing cow milk is similar to that of a dairy goat. Take time to read those sections starting with "Equipment" on page 99. The exceptions and differences are provided below.

- Cows can be milked in the field, in stanchions, in the barn, tied or untied, in open weather or under the protection of a milking shed. The preference is both hers and yours, but some cows are more particular about the ceremony than others.

- A cow does not need a gentle bump at the end of milking each teat. You will know when no more milk exists in her udder as her teats will lay flat.
- To dry up a cow—two months before calving—stop milking her altogether. Do not attempt to wean her off the process or slow down production over a period of days. Her body will stop producing milk the day you stop milking her and after a few days of discomfort she'll absorb the milk left in the udder right back into her body.

Preparing Cattle for the Butcher

Take extra care in the final week of a cow, heifer, steer, or calf's time with you by moving the animal into a pen or stall. Some farmers elect to contain the animal for two weeks and may dramatically increase grain or corn ration during this time. Others prefer to maintain a grass-fed animal and confine the animal for only a few days on the best hay.

Grass-fed cattle—as you'll remember in the introduction to this section—produce beef that is lower in fat and calories and is as tender as the age of the animal affords. Beef finished off on a diet that is largely corn and grain—as many of the old-timers will attest to—is wonderfully marbled and decidedly tender. Whichever route you choose, do not feed cattle for twenty-four hours before butchering, but continue to provide water.

Although throughout this entire book I have touted the farmer's creed, "If you grew it to eat it, you'd better be man enough to kill it," I believe that this job is best left to the professionals. Although countless farmers for hundreds of years have managed the task themselves, the chore is intense. You only need to do it once in your life, just so you can tell others never to attempt it. More importantly however, government regulations throughout the United States and Canada are rigid on the slaughter and butchering of beef at home. Check with officials in your state, region, province, or county to determine your options. Better still, call a local meat processing plant or butcher to arrange for pickup and packaging.

appendices

Recommended Web sites

Chickens and Eggs

American Egg Board
www.aeb.org
US Poultry and Egg Association
www.poultryegg.org
American Poultry Association
http://amerpoultryassn.com
Egg Farmers of Canada
www.eggs.ca
Chicken Farmers of Canada
www.chicken.ca

Goats

American Dairy Goat Association
http://adga.org
American Boer Goat Association
http://abga.org
American Meat Goat Association
www.meatgoats.com
Canadian Goat Society
www.clrc.ca/goats.shtml
Canadian Meat Goat Association
www.canadianmeatgoat.com

Pigs

National Pork Producers Council
www.nppc.org
Canadian Pork Council
www.cpc-ccp.com

Sheep

American Sheep Industry Association
www.sheepusa.org
Canadian Sheep Breeders Association
www.sheepbreeders.ca

Cattle

United States Cattlemen's Association
www.uscattlemen.org
Canadian Cattlemen's Association
www.cattle.ca

General

Animal and Plant Health Inspection Service (America)
www.aphis.usda.gov
United States Animal Health Association
www.usaha.org
American Meat Institute
www.meatami.com
Canadian Food Inspection Agency
http://inspection.gc.ca

Metric Conversions

Unit of Measure	Multiply By:	Converted Unit of Measure
inches	2.54	centimeters
feet	0.3048	meters
miles	1.61	kilometers
square inches	6.452	square centimeters
square feet	0.0929	square meters
acres	0.395	hectares
ounces	28.35	grams
pounds	0.454	kilograms
fluid ounces	29.57	milliliters
gallons	3.785	liters
degrees Fahrenheit	-32 and then multiply by 5/9	degrees Celsius

Glossary

Abscess—A boil under the skin filled with pus.

Afterbirth—Placenta and membranes expelled by a doe after kidding.

Angora—A breed of goat known for excellent fiber.

Antibiotic—Prescribed drug to fight bacterial infections, which may leave residues in the fat or muscle fibers of the animal.

Antibodies—A component of blood that fights disease.

Barn Records—A chart of milk production for each doe or cow. Might also include feeding changes, weather conditions, breeding dates, etc.

Bedding—A natural material used to cover the floor of a farm animal's pen or stall. Wood shavings, straw, waste hay, or shredded paper are standard bedding materials.

Bloat—A distension and swelling of the abdomen as a result of gas buildup.

Bloom—Protective covering of an egg. Unseen once dry.

Buck—Male goat.

Buckling—Male goat under one year old.

Browsing—Eating bushes and woody plants.

Cabrito—The meat of a milk-fed kid.

Cannibalism—A learned habit of chickens, eating another chicken's flesh.

Carrier—An animal that carries disease and infects others, but shows no sign of the disease himself.

Castrate—To remove the testicles of an animal.

Chevon—Goat meat.

Chicken Tractor—a self-contained, movable coop and fenced yard. Most often crafted to house four to six hens.

Coccidiosis—An intestinal disease that causes diarrhea. Coccidiostat is the drug that treats and prevents coccidiosis.

Cockerel—A male bird less than one year old.

Colostrum—Thick, colored milk from a doe or cow that has just given birth. This milk is high in antibodies and is needed by kids or calves for optimum health.

Concentrate—A fortified feed high in nutritional value.

Creep Feeder—A specialty feeder that is built in a manner such that only young may enter and feed.

Crop—A section of a bird's gullet that stores food before digestion.

Cull—To remove inferior animals from the flock or herd.

Dam—An animal's mother.

Dehorn—Surgical operation that removes horns of an adult goat.

Disbud—Removal of the small horn bud of a young animal.

Disbudding Iron—An electric device that burns horn buds from young animals.

Dock—To remove or shorten a tail.

Doe—Female goat.

Doeling—Female goat under the age of one year.

Dual-Purpose or Dual-Purpose Breed—A breed of animal that is exceptional at serving two purposes. Most often pertains to chicken breeds but may also be used for goats, sheep, and cattle.

Electrolytes—A mixture of body salts given to animals suffering from dehydration (usually brought on by scours).

Ewe—A female sheep.

Fleece—Wool from sheep or goats.

Flush—The act of feeding goats and sheep a high ration before breeding to improve probability of conception.

Forage—A combination term used to specify a grass and hay diet as well as allowing animals to pasture and find food on the land.

Free-choice—Always available for the animal's consumption.

Freshen—To rebreed a doe or cow with the intention of producing milk.

Gestation—The time between breeding and birthing.

Grade—Pertaining to an unregistered or crossbred animal.

Grit—Hard materials consumed and used by a bird's gizzard to grind up food for digestion.

Heat—Term used to describe the time a female animal is ready to be bred.

Hen—Female chicken over one year old.

Horn Bud—The beginning of horns.

Kid—A goat under one year old. Also means to birth a goat.

Lamb—Newborn sheep to one year of age.

Legume—A type of plant from the sweet pea family that is found in some hay.

Litter—See Bedding.

Mastitis—An udder inflammation requiring antibiotics.

Mature—Old enough to safely breed.

Meat Birds—Pertaining to chickens. A hybrid or cross (generally with a Cornish breed) known to grow quickly and have a high feed-to-meat conversion.

Milk Stand—Raised platform with a seat for the milker.

Molt—Pertaining to chickens. To lose old feathers before growing new ones.

Mutton—Meat from a mature lamb.

Nesting Box—Box created to accommodate laying hens when laying an egg.

Pecking Order—A highly organized and obeyed social order of chickens.

Pedigree—A certification or registration of an animal's lineage.

Polled—Either born without horns or being a hornless breed.

Poult—A young turkey.

Pullet—Female chicken under the age of one year.

Purebred—An animal that has been registered and whose lineage has been traced for many generations.

Quarantine—To separate one animal from the others for observation or treatment.

Ram—Male sheep. If under one year of age, a ram lamb.

Registration—Animal's ancestry recorded through a recognizable association.

Rotational Grazing—The sequential use of sectioned pasture.

Scours—Severe or persistent diarrhea.

Selenium—Trace mineral required in every animal's diet. Most often gleaned from plants growing in selenium-rich soil. Some areas of North America are now deficient in selenium and therefore it's added to the feed.

Sire—An animal's father.

Stanchions—A device used to hold an animal's head in place during milking.

Straight Run—Mixture of male and female chickens, unsorted, for customer orders.

Strip—Last bit of milk from a goat's udder.

Strip Cup—A cup used for investigation of the first squirt of milk.

Supplement—Extras fed to animals to increase their health.

Vent—The opening of a bird's body for eggs and droppings.

Wean—To stop a particular feeding practice.

Wether—Castrated buck (or buckling) or ram (or ram lamb).

Whey—The remaining liquid when making cheese solids.

Photo Credits

Erin Neese: xiv, 9, 54, 56, 62, 73, 75, 115, 137, 191; Laura Childs: 1, 27, 29, 69, 97, 100, 166; Veronica Childs: 24, 25, 34, 109, 132, 135, 152, 157, back flap; Jacqueline Fouché: 39; Nigel R. Clarke: 51; Franci Strumpfer: 61; Oscar Dahl: 96; Helen Davies: 71; Bas Silderhuis: 122; Ricardo Quintero: 128; Steve Mulford: 130; Luke Miller: 176; Magda Rocio: 180; Stefanie Leuker: 182 ; Gavin Mills: 186; Elmari Briedenhann: 194; Michael Swanson: 214

Page 119: "Slices of goat cheese" by Quinn Dombrowski, https://www.flickr.com/photos/quinnanya/2907545950, is licensed under CC BY-SA 2.0 (https://creativecommons.org/licenses/by-sa/2.0/)

Unless otherwise indicated, photographs are licensed by **Shutterstock.com**.

Barn Records and Forms

Also available at www.KeepingFarmAnimals.com.

CHICKEN
cheat sheet and fast facts

* based on 25 chickens *

Birth Date / /	Breed	Class	Expected Leave / /

Week 1	Week 4	Week 6	Week 18-22	Weeks 23+
90-92°F	75°F	45-80°F ——————————————————————→
15 sq. ft	50 sq. ft.	100 sq. ft. ——————————————————→

←——————————— water: 2 to 4 gallons per day ——————————→

| starter crumble | | layer grower | pre-layer | laying ration |
| 25 lbs/wk ——————————————————————→ | 50 lbs/wk ——→ |

layers start laying - increase light
if raising dual-purpose,
cull the roosters

↑
layers / dual-purpose

meat birds
↓

Week 1	Week 4	Week 8	Week 16
	75°F	45-80°F ————————————————→
15 sq. ft	100 sq. ft. ——————————————————→

←——————————— water: 2 to 4 gallons per day ——————————→

| starter crumble | grower pellets ——→ | finishing grain ——————→ |
| 25 lbs/wk | 50 lbs/wk | 100 lbs/wk ——————————→ |

Date	Notes / Worming / Feed & Medication Changes
/ /	_____
/ /	_____
/ /	_____
/ /	_____

GOAT
breeding and birth record

Doe's Name

Reg. No.

Registry

Date of Breeding   /   /

Buck's Name

Buck's Reg. No.

Buck's Registry

Buck's Owner Name

Address

Buck's Owner Signature

Expected Kid Date   /   /

Actual Birth Date   /   /

Name / ID Kid #1

Sex

Weight

Descriptive features and notes:

Name / ID Kid #2

Sex

Weight

Descriptive features and notes:

Name / ID Kid #3

Sex

Weight

Descriptive features and notes:

GOAT
health docket for

Birth Date / /	Tag/Tattoo/Reg	Registry

Sex	Sire	Dam

Vaccinations:

Date	Vaccination	Veterinarian
/ /		
/ /		
/ /		
/ /		

Worming:

Date	Medication Used	Dosage
/ /		
/ /		
/ /		
/ /		

Weight:

Date	Weight	Feed Changes?
/ /		
/ /		
/ /		
/ /		

Date	Notes / Milk Record / Grain Changes
/ /	
/ /	
/ /	
/ /	
/ /	
/ /	
/ /	
/ /	

GOAT
purchase agreement

Use of this form is at your own discretion and should not be considered legal counsel.

Birth Date / /	Tag/Tattoo/Reg	Registry

Sex	Sire	Dam

Seller's Name	Seller's Address

Buyer's Name	Buyer's Address

Today's Date / /	Amount Received	Goat's Veterinarian

Worming / Medications / Vaccination / Castration / Breeding

Date		Particulars
/ /		
/ /		
/ /		
/ /		

Seller's Disclaimer and Buyer's Responsibilities

_____ , (hereinafter referenced as "Seller"), is making the goat referenced above available to _____ (Buyer) on a "where is, as is" basis, and other than guaranteeing Buyer that said goat is in good health, are free of injury or disease at the date of sale, and that same will breed if provided with the propoer care, environment, and nutrition, Seller makes no other guarantes or warranties, either expressed or implied. Any subsequent claims by Buyer, contesting Seller's representation as to the health, physical condition, or breeding soundness of the subject goat at date of sale must be fully substantiated by a physical examination and applicable medical tests performed by a licensed veterinarian and provided in writing to the Seller.

Applicable registration certificates or registration applications will be provided to Buyer if applicable, within fifteen (15) days of Seller's payment-in-full for the subject purchase, and Seller has confirmed that said payment is in valid funds.

All expenses pertaining to the transportation of the purchased goat from or to the facilities of _____ to or from the Buyer's facilities are the responsibility of the Buyer.

/ /	Seller's Name	Seller's Signature
/ /	Buyer's Name	Buyer's Signature

HEIFER / COW
health, breeding and milk

Birth Date / /	Tag / Name	Breed / Color

Birth Weight	Expected Mature Weight	Sire	Dam

Vaccinations/Medications:

Date	Vaccination	Vet / Clear date
/ /		
/ /		
/ /		
/ /		

Breeding and Calving History:

Heat	Breeding	Expected	Actual Calf	Notes
/ /	/ /	/ /	/ /	
/ /	/ /	/ /	/ /	
/ /	/ /	/ /	/ /	
/ /	/ /	/ /	/ /	

Milking Records:

Date	Quantity	Date	Quantity	Date	Quantity
/ /		/ /		/ /	
/ /		/ /		/ /	
/ /		/ /		/ /	
/ /		/ /		/ /	
/ /		/ /		/ /	
/ /		/ /		/ /	
/ /		/ /		/ /	
/ /		/ /		/ /	
/ /		/ /		/ /	
/ /		/ /		/ /	
/ /		/ /		/ /	
/ /		/ /		/ /	
/ /		/ /		/ /	

PIG
cheat sheet and fast facts

| Birth Date / / | Sex | Name | Expected Leave / / |

| 40 pounds | 60 | 75 | 125 | 220 pounds |

85-90°F   65-70°F

20 sq. ft   40 sq. ft.   75 sq. ft   100 sq. ft.

←—train to electric fence ←→ worm at 10 and 14 weeks

←————————— water: 2 to 4 gallons per day ——————————→

starter feed   grower feed   finisher feed
3 lbs / day   5 ½ lbs / day   7+ lbs / day

HG X HG X L / 400 = WEIGHT

Where HG = Heart Girth and L = Center of Head to Base of Tail
If final equation is less than 150, add 7 pounds.

Date   Notes / Worming Dates / Feed Changes
/ /
/ /
/ /
/ /
/ /
/ /
/ /
/ /

SHEEP
health and maintenance

Birth Date / /	Tag / Name	Breed / Color

Sex	Birth Weight	Sire	Dam

Vaccinations:

Date	Vaccination	Veterinarian
/ /		
/ /		
/ /		
/ /		

Worming:

Date	Medication Used	Dosage
/ /		
/ /		
/ /		
/ /		

Lambing History:

Exposure Date	Lambing Date	Ear Tag Numbers of Lambs
/ /	/ /	
/ /	/ /	
/ /	/ /	
/ /	/ /	

Date	Notes / Weight / Grain Changes
/ /	
/ /	
/ /	
/ /	
/ /	
/ /	
/ /	
/ /	

Index